In Defiance of Death

In Defiance of Death

Exposing the Real Costs of End-of-Life Care

Kenneth A. Fisher, M.D., with Lindsay E. Rockwell, D.O., and Missy Scott

Foreword by Benjamin Brown, M.D.

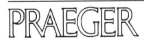

Westport, Connecticut
London

Library of Congress Cataloging-in-Publication Data

Fisher, Kenneth A., 1941–
    In defiance of death : exposing the real costs of end-of-life care / Kenneth A. Fisher ;
with Lindsay E. Rockwell and Missy Scott ; foreword by Benjamin Brown.
        p. ; cm.
    Includes bibliographical references and index.
    ISBN: 978–0–275–99710–6 (alk. paper)
    1. Terminal care—Moral and ethical aspects—United States.   2. Palliative
treatment—Moral and ethical aspects—United States.   3. Death—United
States.   I. Rockwell, Lindsay E.   II. Scott, Missy, 1946–   III. Title.
    [DNLM: 1. Terminal Care—economics—United States.   2. Terminal Care—
ethics—United States.   3. Attitude to Death—United States.   4. Health Policy—
United States.   5. Patient Rights—United States.   6. Terminal Care—legislation
& jurisprudence—United States.   7. Terminally Ill—psychology—United States.
WB 310 F534i 2008]
    R726.8.F62   2008
    179.7—dc22   2007043726

British Library Cataloguing in Publication Data is available.

Library of Congress Catalog Card Number: 2007043726
ISBN: 978–0–275–99710–6

First published in 2008

Praeger Publishers, 88 Post Road West, Westport, CT 06881
An imprint of Greenwood Publishing Group, Inc.
www.praeger.com

Printed in the United States of America

The paper used in this book complies with the
Permanent Paper Standard issued by the National
Information Standards Organization (Z39.48-1984).

10 9 8 7 6 5 4 3 2 1

To the many patients I have observed over the years, who were the victims of inappropriate care, especially at the end of their lives.

To the art of medicine; practiced with science, judgment, and compassion.

To my wife. Together we have the gift of love. No man is better than the woman he loves believes him to be.

And to our children, who share our love and concern for humankind.

Contents

Figures and Tables

Figures

Tables

Foreword: The Art of Medicine

There was an idea called "being present" when I went from college to medical school. Perhaps it grew out of the coping that people had to do when the world was changing so dramatically in the 1960s and 1970s. The phrase meant you tried to put yourself in the other person's world. It wasn't about expressing your own opinion in response to what they were saying. Being present was and is about letting yourself listen to another, to the extent that you see things from their point of view.

This wasn't what I was taught in medical school at all. Medical school was about having arrived at the "Club." We spoke another language from our patients. We knew what they didn't know, and we could tell them what to do. We were in control. The patient presented some facts to us, which we reframed to fit our knowledge. We added facts of our own. Then we told them what to do.

Fortunately, that wasn't the only approach among my young colleagues. But the attitude irritated me disproportionately. I didn't like the uniform white coats that distinguished us. I didn't want to sit across a desk from the person whose insides I needed to understand. Most of all, I wanted to hear what they thought of their illness.

It's fascinating how much patients will tell you, if you give them the chance. Of course, some people go on and on, almost avoiding the important issues. Some people test the doctor to see how much she or he knows. Some people hide important points until the end of the interview or until the next interview. However, most people have crucial insights into their medical predicament that help the doctor.

I learned long ago that patients would usually tell me not only what their problem was but also how they would like to approach it. This is paramount these days. A doctor can be very aggressive by ordering every test and using every intervention possible. This may be what my next patient wants. However this patient may also have a high deductible and want my best opinion about how to save money and still manage her headaches, back pain, or numbness well. She may have friends with whom she has been discussing her problems and has come to the office with preconceived intentions. She may have specific fears that she is afraid to verbalize, which are not in my imagination at all.

For me, it has always been important to use the person's wisdom, fears, intuition, and social and economic situations in my plan. In fact, I don't usually have only one plan. I often have several plans that are contingent upon the person's reaction to the various options. This takes some to and fro in the conversation. I have to hear what's between the words. I may need to create pregnant pauses. I may need to venture an idea on a hunch, and then be ready to accept being off the mark if the patient doesn't connect with that idea.

What does this take? It takes willingness to be in another person's world. It takes being present. It is very hard to be present in modern medicine.

First there were the lawyers. The threat of going to court to defend one's actions is a powerful motivator for a doctor to think inside the box and to order more objective tests than to use subjective judgment. It seems that if I, as the doctor, stay within the protocols, standards, and other cookbooks of medicine, the chances of my being brought to court will be lessened. Actually, however, this turns out not to be true. Malpractice suits are more or less likely based upon the personal relationship the doctor has with the patient. Nevertheless, the malpractice threat creates a very real tension that affects styles of practice and the expression of feelings and ideas between doctor and patient.

More recently, industrial business models have affected medicine. The flow of patients through an office or a hospital is likened to an assembly line. In the office, doctors are pressed to address only one of the patient's problems and move them through. In the hospital, the trend is not for the patients to be cared for by their doctor, but by a series of doctors who do not have the time or perhaps even the interest to be present with them. You will learn later in this book about money as a motivation in healthcare. Unfortunately this can be true for physicians; however, it is the norm for people who oversee physicians.

Administrators of hospitals, doctors' offices, and insurance companies focus upon similarities among patients and medical problems for more uniform billing purposes and economies of scale. Consequently, systems of diagnosis and treatment are arranged to handle patients' most common issues. At the same time, each patient knows how unique his or her entire situation is. With the business model, patients can rest assured only that their typical problems will be addressed and that the common aspects of their situations will be understood. For those who assess and report on healthcare quality, the focus is upon easily measured parameters. However, the patient's perception of quality of care may depend upon aspects that are not easily measurable.

I work as a family physician. We are paid by the number of patients we care for, not by the number of problems we handle. If a patient comes to our office with a single problem, such as ear pain with no complicating issues, we are paid $X.

The next patient may come in for a cold; however, he may also be very depressed due to several terrible things happening in his life recently. He knows, and

I know, that this has played a role in becoming ill and will affect his ability to cope with the illness. I also recognize that this is an important medical issue of its own. Shall I tell him I don't have the time to listen to his story, to address his emotional condition?

What if my third patient has done well enough to reach the age of eighty-five? She may have seven serious chronic illnesses that are in a state of flux, and three non–life-threatening health issues that are, nevertheless, very important to her getting through each day. She may not speak very fast due to her age, and she may talk about events and opinions that are not medically relevant. She might be confused and need a family member to talk for her, a family member who is not with her today. She might not speak English well. She might have had her insurance changed recently or be in the Medicare Part D doughnut hole and need all her meds changed to different but similar ones. I might not be able to tell which medicines she takes regularly and which ones she doesn't even have at home.

When I present an approach to one of the problems presented by these patients, they want and need an explanation of the problem, the various other diagnoses that could be involved, how best to work it up, what the complications of working it up might be, what medicines they will need, what side effects these medicines may have, what interactions with their other medicines may occur, and what red flags to watch for with the condition or medicines that would necessitate them calling back early. Then we can start on how their family members may respond to this plan and these medicines. We can talk about how they are going to pay for this. We should review all these details because they are complicated and hard to remember.

Then we go on to problem number two.

When we see a patient with multiple problems such as this, modern insurance, federal or private, pays our office approximately one and one half times $X, the amount reimbursed for the simple cold. This is poor incentive indeed for me to listen long and hard to find the most effective, and cost-effective, approach for each one of the patient's conditions and communicate them well.

Another more subtle, yet I believe powerful phenomenon occurs when doctor and patient sit together for longer than business practices recommend. When people feel listened to in depth, they start healing themselves. Perhaps as they listen to themselves, they start to do their own observation and planning. Perhaps untold parts of the psyche become free from anger and anxiety and can then shift to work on what they already know they need to do. Perhaps some sort of energy exchanges between doctor and patient. I can't claim to know how exactly it works, but I have watched over and over again as people become their own best ally in the struggle to heal or cope appropriately with their illness, when they get sufficient connection with the physician.

I had one professor who was a mentor in medical school who told me that people come to us, the doctors, so that we will think. That's where he stopped. He wanted us to think hard. We certainly need to think about all we learned in medical school. We also need to think about who the person is, facing us in the gown, who is ill and perhaps feeling vulnerable. We need to come out of ourselves to try to walk in their shoes for a while. We also need to hear our own intuition. And then we need to use our best intellectual abilities to help them navigate the healthcare world with their medical issues. This is how the art and science of medicine mix.

As part of my current practice, I care for many elderly people. Having practiced for a few decades, I am heading down the "getting older" road myself. This is where my parents have already gone. As they became ill, I spent much time with my siblings sorting out how we felt about each of my parents' different situations before they ultimately died. Professionally, some of my favorite stories in medicine are about the times when people are close to dying. I've always felt that a "good death" was every bit as touching, meaningful, and even awesome (in the original sense of the word) as a birth.

When I get ready to die, I will want the caretakers around me not to be thinking about what procedure will improve my lab numbers. Rather, I want them to think about what I am experiencing, hoping for, and what my family understands. I know that my doctor will not spend as much time with me as the nurses and other caretakers. However, when my doctor is next to me, I want her or him to be present with me. I want them to think outside of the cookbook. I know death will come. I would like to greet it in my own way.

Benjamin Brown, M.D.

Preface

Every society in history has shown reverence for the dead. But what happens to a society that lacks reverence for the dying, and does not honor death as a natural process? What happens to a society that decides that the rights of the family or others, who cannot or will not deal with the reality of the situation, supersede the right of the dying person to a dignified and loving death?

The results are catastrophic! A compassionate and caring profession loses its way and uses its skills and techniques inappropriately. With time, this attitude spreads throughout the profession, with hundreds of thousands lingering in nursing homes. When death nears, they are repeatedly shuttled off to acute care or specialty hospitals for "rescue," then returned to the nursing home to suffer a lingering, disfiguring death. The profession loses its perspective on the use of technologies, adding great expense to the society, with little or no gain for patients and their families.

Great institutions of learning become mesmerized by the procedures and the income produced, using their intellectual force, in many cases, to generate income with little or no gain for the patient and loss for the society. Instead of being a model for the wise mix of procedures and compassion, they become the purveyors of the inappropriate use of this technology or that procedure. The costs to society become so great that no matter how much more is spent on medical care, the results keep getting worse. As businesses and corporations try to recoup, some of the astronomical cost of healthcare for their employees and retirees, manufactured goods are priced out of the global market, jobs are lost, and millions go without ready access to healthcare.

The society I am writing about is that of the United States. I have seen the drift of a noble profession that has lost its way, causing untold grief in the name of medical care. The most extreme example of this wayward behavior is keeping the cardiovascular-respiratory system functioning with machines and drugs, as the patient develops massive skin ulcers, decaying digits, and an irretrievable loss of the cerebral cortex—the part of the brain that is the source of our humanness. I have watched a legal system make decisions that perpetuate this hideous behavior by referring to laws in the abstract instead of dealing with the individual case of a human being and its unique medical facts.

I have seen medical students choose the more lucrative and emotionally less taxing specialties to avoid dealing with this human tragedy that occurs daily in every medical facility in the nation. I have seen the funding for the education of our young compromised by the irresponsible use of resources by the medical profession. I have witnessed my own medical society remain silent on the issues of the permanent vegetative state, our responsibility as physicians to make the best use of both medical and financial resources, and the lack of support for the primary care physician who does not hawk procedures but rather thinking and compassion.

After forty years of watching the profession I love go astray, I had to write this book. My intent is to lay out the situation as it stands today and offer solutions that could steer things back to a strong, healthy course. It is my hope that this book will inspire a spirited national debate, starting at the grass roots and spreading to the halls of Congress. I have great faith in the American people to rally to a cause, and few among us have not had some kind experience with end-of-life care as it exists today. Perhaps that combination of hope and faith will lead to meaningful reforms that will return the dying process to what it really is—an honored, natural passage of life.

Kenneth A. Fisher, M.D.

Acknowledgments

I thank Nicholas Philipson, my original editor at Praeger, who saw the merit of this project. I thank Jeff Olson, my present editor at Praeger, who has helped refine this work.

As a child in grammar school English, I usually received high marks for ideas but poor grades for spelling, grammar, and word flow. I have not changed. I knew if I was going to get my ideas across to the public, I needed help with grammar and the rhythm of my writing to better convey my message. I thus sought help; Lindsay Rockwell and Missy Scott have contributed to this book so that my idea flow is coherent on the page. However, I am the "I" speaking in the book.

CHAPTER 1

Dying in America Today

It was early May when Nora Downes died. A soft spring breeze rippled the curtains at the window of her bedroom in the house she had shared with her husband of nearly sixty years. He was at her side, holding her hand. Her children and grandchildren were all there with her, and, saddened as they were, they were grateful for her peaceful passage. They were also grateful for the support of the hospice workers who had not only helped with her care during her final illness, but also made sure she was physically comfortable and in no pain.

On the same day, across town at the county hospital, Jim Wallace was entering yet another week in the Intensive Care Unit after being transferred from the nursing home where he had lived in declining health for nearly two years. At seventy-eight, following a massive stroke, he was on life support and showing no signs of recovery. He didn't seem aware of his family during their limited, short visits, and the team of physicians caring for him had suggested that discontinuing life support might be appropriate. The family, however, felt he might "come around," and refused. The physician's hands were tied at that point, and so his saga continues.

Studies show that 90 percent of us would rather die peacefully like Mrs. Downes, surrounded by family and friends, as comfortable as possible. The reality is that nearly 80 percent of us will end up like Mr. Wallace,[1] languishing in a hospital, often in an expensive Intensive Care Unit, with very little contact with family and friends.[2] In my 40-plus years of medical practice, I have seen far more scenarios like Mr. Wallace than Mrs. Downes. I have come to see dying in America as an often protracted medicalized techno-process that is hurtful to the patients and their families, and ultimately to the very fabric of our society.

There was a time in our not-so-distant past when you could walk into a room full of first-year medical students, ask how many of them had ever been around a dead body before they came to med school, and just about every hand in the class would go up. Most older people or terminally ill people died at home, and those that died in a hospital did so with few, if any, life-prolonging interventions. Family members were generally there at their passing, and they usually took part in their care during the last phase of the dying person's life, especially those who died at home. Wakes brought family and friends together to celebrate the life of the deceased loved one and to mourn their passing. Wakes were usually held at home, with the deceased present and at the center of everything, and sometimes went on for days. Death was a natural part of life.

Today, ask that same question to a first-year medical school class, and very few hands will go up. Yet we still have a fascination with death. It's always big news in the media, and the funeral industry is booming. But how did we get so far away from the simple truth that death is a natural process of life to the point that dying has become a nightmare for so many patients and their families? Is it a spiritual issue? A societal cycle? Perhaps an economic trend fueled by the growth of medical advances and technology? Or even a crisis of leadership within the medical community itself? It is most likely a subtle evolution of all of those things together; so subtle, in fact, that we were unable to see it coming. Now the problem has become too enormous to ignore.

Modern technology fuels the ability to stave off death and the fear that surrounds it. Pharmaceutical ads on television tout the wonders of the latest new drug. The mainstream news media frequently describes additional "miracles" of medicine and their potential, life-saving positive impact. We have created a vast medical enterprise to fight death.

No wonder patients and families are bewildered when they are told that dying is inevitable. As a result, physicians often find themselves in the awkward predicament of being asked to prolong a life that may no longer be viable because the body is still breathing and sustains a pulse, but not much else. For some patients, whose illnesses are really beyond treatment, hospitals can become halls of trauma, frustration, and bureaucracy, rather than sanctuaries of healing or hospice.

An honest, open dialogue between doctors and patients who are dying and their families can help restore the balance. At the same time, we must examine closely—with an eye toward meaningful reform—the ethical, social, and political issues that have brought us to this point.

THE WORKING DEFINITION OF DEATH

Each of us has our own thoughts about death and what it means. We physicians, however, must go by the current medical/legal definition of brain death. I personally do not agree with this definition and think it should be changed. However, it will be helpful for you to know the definition and keep it in mind as you read this book.

The definition of brain death was created in 1968 in response to the need to create a more humane definition of death and to help procure organs for transplant. An ad hoc committee of the Harvard Medical School developed guidelines based on the premise that, with the loss of total brain activity, coma was irreversible and further care futile.[3] These guidelines have been accepted worldwide as the standard. But this definition left open a gray area—you can lose use of the more sensitive cerebral cortex, while maintaining use of the brain stem, which allows such things as respiration and other bodily functions. This causes what we now call the persistent vegetative state, as in the Terri Schiavo case.[4] Is the patient "dead" or not? Medical societies have remained silent during national healthcare debates on this subject, so any national discourse on this difficult issue takes place largely in the absence of medical science.

Today we know so much more about brain function than we did in 1968. Neurological, biological, and physiological evidence points to the cerebral cortex as the location of "self," or personhood. It is the thinking, feeling, speaking, motion-controlling part of the brain. When a patient has lost the function of the cerebral cortex, you may see what looks like a person, but what we call "human" is absent. The *person* is gone. Yet we still make decisions about end-of-life care based on what is an outmoded definition. We will explore the role of this definition further in Chapter 2.

HOW WE HAVE EVOLVED TO THIS POINT

Several crucial events, and their ensuing consequences over the years, have led us to where we are today.

1. After World War II, the United States embarked on a medical research program unparalleled in human history. The National Institutes of Health, pharmaceutical companies, foundations, and citizen groups like the March of Dimes funded this work, which was and still is primarily focused on the mechanisms of disease and their treatments. Many of the problems we have today with end-stage chronic illness are a result of the success of these programs and the ability to prolong life.

2. When cardiopulmonary resuscitation (CPR) was introduced in the 1960s, the average hospital patient population was much younger than it is today, so the policy of CPR by default often led to successful outcomes. This is not the case today, and, in the absence of a do not resuscitate order, routine CPR often adds to the suffering of a dying patient with no reasonable hope of a positive outcome.

3. With the advent of Medicare and Medicaid in 1965, Congress adopted a fee-for-service payment schedule. Payments for procedures were reimbursed at a higher rate than the more difficult-to-define areas, such as critical thinking, time spent speaking to patients, and preventive care. In the 1980s, Medicare began reimbursing hospitals using diagnostic-related groups (DRGs), and now other insurers are using similar systems. DRGs are patient classification systems that group patients according to diagnosis and treatment for the purpose of setting uniform payment rates for hospital care. The goal was more

cost-effective care. However, payment for procedures and intensive care are still reimbursed at a much higher rate than physician fees for service (see Figure 1.1).

4. As Medicare and Medicaid budgets have grown, the response has been across-the-board cuts instead of dealing with specific high-cost problems such as end-of-life care. Consequently, there is now a greater emphasis on billable procedures, and more emphasis on admitting patients to Intensive Care Units (ICUs) even if these are not beneficial or appropriate for the end-of-life patient. On the losing end is primary care, the very heart of medicine, as physicians have less time to spend with patients and families. Hospital physicians experience this time crunch as well, so it's no wonder that doctor/patient communication is minimal.

5. Medicare, the major source of funds for graduate medical education, has cut funding to the point that hospitals are receiving less than they did in 1996. The same is true of funding for subspecialty training DME (direct medical education reimbursement).[5] Academic medical centers (big teaching hospitals) have been forced to significantly increase the volume of patient care to prevent deficits and cover their high fixed costs. That means less time for teaching and helping medical students learn the *art* of medicine: obtaining a history, physical exam skills, getting to know a patient more personally, critical thinking, and learning when testing and technology are appropriate and when they are not. Clinical teachers are pressured to increase their billable patient loads, meaning less and less time for teaching. With so much more emphasis on profitability, medical schools often have a harsh commercial air about them, with students hearing as much about throughput, market share, units of service, and the bottom line as they do about preventive care, relief of suffering, patient well-being, and compassion.[6]

6. Patient autonomy means that patients have the right to refuse appropriate therapy. However, many people have interpreted this to mean that patients have the right to insist on and receive inappropriate therapy. The ramifications of this interpretation are covered in depth in Chapter 2.

7. The organized medical community has been very reluctant to enter public debates on controversial end-of-life subjects like the persistent vegetative state. Consequently, individual physicians have little support or guidance in dealing rationally with these profound medical dilemmas. In many instances, the courts make the decisions, without appropriate and critical medical input.

8. Facing the specter of lawsuits, doctors and hospitals are more apt to overdo treatment in end-of-life situations. This is particularly true of larger teaching hospitals, which have a much larger array of technological diagnostic and treatment procedures.

Figure 1.1. Diagnostic Related Group (DRG) Payment System.

This is an example of a DRG form showing the costly, and ultimately futile treatment of a patient at the end of her life. You don't need to understand the "doctor speak" to see that this patient had multiple health problems, and the procedures that were performed may have actually created more.

Hypothetical Case

A seventy-eight-year-old woman with long-standing diabetes and coronary artery disease is admitted to the hospital because of severe diarrhea, secondary to antibiotics for lower leg cellulitis. She develops an acute myocardial infarction (non-ST wave elevation), or a severe heart attack, receives cardiac catheterization with stenting, and develops acute renal failure requiring dialysis and bleeds eight units of blood from the catheterization site. She requires intensive care for shortness of breath, and after eight days in the unit, she dies. Her total hospital costs amounted to approximately $20,000. If a tracheotomy had been performed the payment under other procedures would have been about another $100,000.

Medicare DRG:
557   Percutaneous Cardiovascular Procedure with drug-eluting stent with a major cardiovascular diagnosis.
         CMS wt.   2.7616   A/LOS 4.1   G/LOS 3.0

Principal Diagnosis:
41041   Acute myocardial infarction, inferior wall, initial episode of care

Secondary Diagnosis:
41401   Coronary atherosclerosis of native coronary vessel
 9961   Mechanical complication of vascular device/implant/graft
 5849   Acute renal failure, unspecified
25080   Diabetes mellitus with specified manifestation, type II or unspecified type, not stated as uncontrolled
 6826   Cellulitis and abscess of leg, except foot
78791   Diarrhea

Principal Procedure:
 0066   Percutaneous transluminal coronary angioplasty (PTCA) or coronary atherectomy

Other Procedures:
 3723   Combined right and left heart cardiac catheterization
 3607   Insertion of drug-eluting coronary artery stent(s)
 0041   Procedure on two vessels
 0046   Insertion of two vascular stents
 3895   Venous catheterization for renal dialysis
 3995   Hemodialysis
 9903   Transfusion of whole blood
 9604   Insertion of endotracheal tube
 9672   Continuous mechanical ventilation for 96 consecutive hours or more

I certify that the narrative descriptions of the principal and secondary diagnoses and the major procedures performed are accurate and complete to the best of my knowledge.

Source: Adapted from www.ahd.com/pps.html with help from the finance department at Bronson Methodist Hospital, Kalamazoo, MI.

THE BURGEONING COST OF HEALTHCARE AND THE NATIONAL ECONOMY

Many people like to crow about the United States having the best healthcare system in the world, and much of the public believes that. The truth is that we have an outrageously expensive healthcare system that spends more per person on healthcare than any other nation in the world—a total of $1.4 trillion a year as of 2001[7]—yet our overall health outcomes are poor in comparison to other developed nations,[8] and over 46 million people do not have health insurance.[‡]

Medicare reimbursement practices that pay more for procedures than a physician's time, skewed interpretations of patient autonomy, and physicians' fear of lawsuits are more often than not the culprits in poor end-of-life care.

In disability-adjusted life expectancy (DALE), the United States is 24th behind many industrialized and non-industrialized countries.[9] In health-adjusted life expectancy (HALE), the United States is 29th with an average of 69.3 years.[10] Previous studies indicate the United States to be in the bottom fourth of industrialized countries in health indicators such as life expectancy and infant mortality.[11]

A big chunk of that high price tag is inappropriate end-of-life care. As the Baby Boomers reach age 70 and beyond, the costs to our society will become astronomical if we continue to practice our present style of end-of-life care. According to a Census Bureau Special Report,[12] the oldest of the 78 million Baby Boomers started turning 60 in 2006 at a rate of nearly 8,000 a day. It's only a matter of time before those numbers begin to significantly impact healthcare in general, and end-of-life care in particular. According to a 2002 U.S. General Accounting Office report, "Long-term care spending from all public and private sources, which was about $137 billion for persons of all ages in 2000, will increase dramatically in the coming decades as the baby boom generation ages. Spending on long-term care services just for the elderly is projected to increase at least two-and-a-half times and could nearly quadruple in constant dollars to $379 billion by 2050, according to some estimates."[13] Table 1.1 illustrates the steep climb in the number of older people in the coming years.

One study on this topic found that medical expenditures (1996 dollars) for patients 65 years and older were $7,365 for nonterminal years, and $37,581 during the last year of life.[14] Another found costs in the last year of life averaged $28,201 with about one-third in the last month before death.[15] Only patients with cancer using hospice had lower costs. Yet another study found that in California and Massachusetts, medical expenditures for the last year of life averaged $31,550 for patients 65–74 years of age and $21,800 for those 85 years and older.[16] Although the $21,800 is about three times the nonfatal year found in the previous study, the $10,000 difference is probably due to physicians, patients, and families more readily accepting the impending death of a much older loved one, and a greater willingness to use palliative or hospice care, rather than more expensive procedures and treatment.

Interestingly enough, avoidable deaths have been in steep decline over the past 50 years, while unavoidable death rates have had only a small decrease.[17]

[‡](To read more, see Appendix 8, "What Cannot Be Said on Television about Health Care.")

Table 1.1. Projections of U.S. Elderly Population

Year	Mean Age	Population 65+ (in millions)	% of Population 65+	% Increase from 2000 in 65+ Population
2000	36.5	34.71	12.6	—
2005	37.2	36.17	12.6	4.2
2010	37.8	39.41	13.2	13.5
2020	39.0	53.22	16.5	53.3
2030	39.9	69.38	20.0	99.9
2040	40.3	75.23	20.3	116.8
2050	40.3	78.86	20.0	127.2

U.S. Department of Health and Human Services, Aging of the Population, *Changing Demographics and the Implications for Physicians, Nurses, and Other Health Workers, 2003.*

Doesn't this tell us something very profound? We must learn when death is unavoidable, and then switch from highly technical attempts at hopeless curative care to palliative/hospice care.

According to a report by the Henry J. Kaiser Foundation and the Health Research and Education Group, rapidly rising healthcare costs could eventually bankrupt the national economy.[18] Even though the increase in healthcare costs from the spring of 2005 to the spring of 2006 was modest in a historical perspective, it was still twice as great as the increase in wages. We are now spending 17 percent of Gross Domestic Product (GDP) on healthcare, and that's a big financial drag on both businesses and employees. The high cost of employee healthcare coverage here at home plays a big role in the decisions of many companies to outsource labor overseas. The financial burden continues to increase for employees as well. Covered employees still pay 27 percent of the costs of their health insurance, but their monthly payments have increased from $129 in 1999 to $248 per month in 2006. No data were presented on how much end-of-life care contributes to these costs, but the data presented in upcoming chapters of this book suggest it is a significant amount.

How much longer can the national economy stand the pressures of skyrocketing healthcare costs?

In a letter to President Bush, the Business Roundtable said, "Health care costs are the top cost pressures restraining companies' ability to grow." Although the Roundtable made many suggestions, they did not mention or did not grasp the significance of end-of-life costs.[19]

I live in Michigan, so am very familiar with the economic woes of the three big automakers here. General Motors is a classic example of the devastating effects of rising healthcare costs.

The Impact of Healthcare Costs on General Motors

Retiree health benefits cost GM $3.6 billion in 2005, more than two-thirds of its total health spending.[20] The fraction spent on end-of-life care was not discussed. The question of whether GM could have seen considerable savings, or whether these patients and their families would have received better care in a hospice setting for end-of-life treatment was not addressed. Healthcare costs are not entirely responsible for the GM downsizing from 600,000 employees in 1979 to an estimated 125,000 in 2005–2006, but it certainly is a contributing factor. Inappropriate end-of- life care comprises a significant portion of those costs. The other two other "legacy" domestic automakers have similar problems. An interesting side note: Approximately $1,500 is tacked on to the price of every GM car and truck just to cover healthcare costs.[§]

IMPACT OF AGGRESSIVE, NONBENEFICIAL END-OF-LIFE CARE

The Public

A survey of family members and significant others of 1,578 deceased patients was conducted to determine the quality of physical and emotional support to the pa-tient, whether decision making was shared, if the dying person was treated with respect, if the families' emotional needs were met, and whether care was coor-dinated.[21] Most patients (67 per-cent) died in an institution, while 16 percent died in hospice care. Those dying at home with hospice were felt to have received excellent care more frequently than those dying in other situations, such as hospitals or nursing homes.

Patients, families, physicians, physicians in training, and our society all suffer the consequences of poor end-of-life care.

Medical Schools

Options for palliative care are not currently covered extensively in the train-ing of new physicians in end-of-life care. (Palliative care is supportive care aimed at making the patient as comfortable as possible by controlling symptoms and minimizing pain. In end-of-life situations, it should become the focus when cura-tive treatment is no longer effective.) Using the palliative education assessment tool (PEAT) for medical education,[22] New York medical schools have enhanced the palliative care content in their curricula. There is now a full curriculum for

[§](To read more, see Appendix 7, "Aging Baby Boom Generation Will Increase De-mand and Burden on Federal and State Budgets.")

teaching palliative care to medical students,[23] and it should become a part of every prospective doctor's training.**

Resident Physicians

A review of the literature from 1966 to 2005 found that residents were unprepared to handle patient end-of-life decisions and misinterpreted do not resuscitate (DNR) orders and the concept of nonbeneficial care. The residents found that the end-of-life decision-making process did not reflect in real-world practice what they had been taught in medical school.[24]

Practicing Physicians

A 2004 survey of 1,236 physicians from different specialties asked how they rated their training in ten competencies in the care of patients with chronic illness, geriatric syndromes, chronic pain, nutrition, developmental milestones, end-of-life care, psychological issues, patient education, assessment of caregiver needs, coordination of services, and interdisciplinary teamwork. Most physicians thought their training in these areas was inadequate.[25]

In another study of practicing physicians,[26] the three greatest barriers to appropriate end-of-life care were:

1. Physicians' reluctance to make referrals to hospice.
2. Physicians' lack of understanding about the availability and usefulness of hospice.
3. The association of hospice with death.

Dr. Kenneth I. Shine, a cardiologist and past president of the National Institute of Medicine, sums things up beautifully in his editorial in the *Annals of Internal Medicine*.[27] He points out that

- The greater the availability of hospital resources and physicians (specialists and subspecialists), the more they will be used, whether they provide any benefit to the patient or not.
- Medical societies should begin to teach their members and the public that in end-of-life situations, appropriate care is not more technological care, but rather palliative care.
- Care that adds no value should be avoided, and could save about one-third of our total healthcare costs.

** (To read more, see Appendix 5, "American Medical Education 100 Years after the Flexner Report.")

- Physicians should lead in this effort to provide appropriate care because the government and insurance carriers are not equipped to perform this task.
- Physicians must engage and educate the public, explaining to them that this is about better care, not rationing.

MY UNSCIENTIFIC BUT REVEALING SURVEY

As part of the research for this book, I decided to see what people had to say about their experiences with end-of-life care. I designed some simple questionnaires for different groups of people—like families, nurses, doctors, and so on—and created a Web site so that people could tell their stories (www.dying-in-america. com). You will also find the questionnaires in Appendix 1. You may find it interesting to fill out the questionnaire that best suits you and then fill it out again after you read the book to see how your views may have changed. Chapter 9 deals with the results of the study in more detail, but the overwhelming message is that end-of-life care is often unnecessarily expensive; puts dying patients through needless, hopeless procedures; fails to discuss palliative care or hospice; and needs serious reform.

CHAPTER 2

Roots of the Problem: The Patient Self-Determination Act, Advance Directives, and the Americans with Disabilities Act

As we shall see, it's not hard to find the roots of many problems in our approach to end-of-life care.

GENESIS OF THE PATIENT SELF-DETERMINATION ACT (PSDA)

Two very high-profile cases—one in 1975 and the other in 1983—prompted the debates that led to the passage of the Patient Self-Determination Act in 1990. It went into effect in 1991. As you read through these two cases, keep in mind the working definition of brain death mentioned in Chapter 1.

Case 1: Karen Ann Quinlan

In 1975, 21-year-old Karen Ann Quinlan had a transient episode of lack of oxygen supply to her cerebral cortex, causing permanent loss of function. Her brain stem, however, was still functional, and thus she did not meet the criteria of brain death. Technology kept Karen's bodily functions intact: stable blood pressure, active digestion system, and adequate kidney function. In the absence of cerebral cortex function, the person Karen Ann Quinlan was gone. Karen's father wanted to continue administration of nutrition and water, but discontinue artificial respiration. Her physician, the local prosecutor, and the New Jersey attorney general opposed his wishes. The New Jersey trial court denied the father's appointment as legal guardian and ruled that the attending physician and currently accepted medical standards should prevail. The New Jersey Supreme Court reversed the trial court and appointed Karen's father as guardian. She was weaned from the respirator but was given nutrition and water. Her body slowly deteriorated, and she ceased to exist ten years later.

Case 2: Nancy Cruzan

In 1983, 25-year-old Nancy Cruzan sustained serious injuries in an automobile accident and was resuscitated. However, due to inadequate oxygen to her brain, she lost cerebral cortical function, but retained brain stem activity. Like Karen Quinlan, Nancy's bodily functions were maintained, but Nancy the person had ceased to exist. Her parents, knowing their child would not want to be kept alive artificially while slowly decaying away, sought to have her feeding tube and other support measures stopped.

Because she was in a state hospital, the case landed in the Missouri Supreme Court. The court agreed that a person had the right to refuse treatment, but did not feel Nancy had made her wishes "clear and convincing."[1] The court decided that this was not a case of the right to die but the right of others to take her life.

In my opinion, the court's finding that the issue was the right of others to take her life was flawed. She, in fact, had no *life* to take. In 1990 the U.S. Supreme Court heard the case and did codify the right of a competent individual to refuse any life-prolonging treatment. In the case of "incompetent" people, a state could insist on clear proof of a person's preference.[2]

This decision was made on legal grounds and with little attention to medical knowledge. The Supreme Court sent the case back to the Missouri Supreme Court, which finally did allow the support services to be removed. Nancy's body quickly ceased to exist.

In response to the above two cases, with input from a presidential commission, Congress passed on November 5, 1990, as a part of the Omnibus Budget Reconciliation Act, the Patient Self-Determination Act. It went into effect on December 1, 1991. This act stated that patients have the right under state law to create advance directives stipulating what they wish done in an end-of-life situation.

PROBLEMS WITH THE PSDA

Before the ink was dry on the bill, medical ethicists and others anticipated many of the problems that would actually appear later. The most serious prediction, and one that has come to be, is that the act places the physician in the position of taking orders about treatment from those without medical knowledge. Kevin O'Rourke, Director of the Center for Health Care Ethics, St. Louis University Medical Center, felt that the PSDA used a sledgehammer approach in a delicate situation:

> Potentially, the most serious ethical issue resulting from PSDA is the implied assumption that physicians are simply to carry out the wishes of the proxy. Physicians must listen to the patient/proxy to learn as clearly as possible what the patient does and does not want, but they ultimately must do what is medically appropriate for the patient. Patient wishes must be interpreted in light of medical knowledge.[3]

As time went on, others came to see that the PSDA had not significantly in-creased the use of written advance care documents, nor had it increased discus-sion between physicians and patients regarding end-of-life issues.[4] It contributed to the illusion that death is an option, and that life can be prolonged indefinitely. The choice paradigm (patient autonomy) presents options that are not real, such as the option of not dying of a terminal illness. It is in these circumstances where the struggle between hope and reality may become not only heart-wrenching but also a source of great contention among family members as well as between family and medical staff who are attempting to encourage the more realistic view. The most positive end-of-life experiences had by both patients and families are those in which all are able and willing to accept death as the final stage of life.[5] In an article in the *Annals of Internal Medicine*, Henry S. Perkins, MD wrote:

> Advance directives promise patients a say in their future care, but actually have had little effect. Many experts blame problems with completion and implementation, but the advance directive concept itself may be funda-mentally flawed. Advance directives simply presuppose more control over future care than is realistic. Medical crises cannot be predicted in detail, making most prior instructions difficult to adapt, irrelevant, or even mis-leading. Furthermore, many proxies either do not know patients' wishes or do not pursue those wishes effectively. Thus, unexpected problems arise often to defeat advance directives. Because advance directives offer only limited benefit, advance care planning should emphasize not the comple-tion of directives but the emotional preparation of patients and families for future crises. The existentialist Albert Camus might suggest that physicians should warn patients and families that momentous, unforeseeable decisions lie ahead. Then, when the crisis hits, physicians should provide guidance; should help make decisions despite the inevitable uncertainties; should share responsibility for those decisions; and, above all, should courageously see patients and families through the fearsome experience of dying.[6]

The PSDA, in its attempt to provide for patient autonomy, oversimplified the complex dynamics of the dying process. When used thoughtfully, and with sound medical judgment, life-saving measures engender and restore faith in medical capabilities, and they offer second chances to patients and families. If, however, when physicians use those same measures in a situation with no chance of recov-ery, then there is enormous potential to do more harm than good.

Another vital yet overlooked aspect of the PSDA is the inherent role of com-munication between the medical providers and the patient and family in the midst of challenging emotional circumstances. Conversations about death and dying occur rarely. In the glare of our current medical culture, intensive care units, oncology units, and fluorescent-laden medical wards, an "appropriate death" is impossible without continuous guidance and support from physicians, nurses, discharge planners, and hospital support staff. Each member plays a pivotal role in the experience of dying. Each must be embraced as we consider reconfiguration of responsibilities and open lines of communication.

Distorting the Concept of Patient Autonomy in the Absence of Advance Directives

The PSDA requires that Medicare/Medicaid provider facilities inform patients of their rights, under their state's laws, to make decisions about their medical care, including the right to refuse care and to formulate an advance directive.[7] There is a significant difference between refusing or limiting care and directing care. There are times when a physician knows there is no hope for recovery, but families or guardians refuse to accept this reality. In the absence of an advance directive, the physician often becomes a kind of technician, taking orders from families or guardians and, in some cases, the courts.

In this regard, people have become consumers of medical services in the same way they are consumers of handbags and golf clubs. This sense of consumerism is clearly illustrated in the case of Baby K.[8] Baby K was born with only a brain stem and without the cerebral cortex, the human part of her brain. The courts supported the mother in her efforts to keep the baby alive on life support against the recommendations of the medical team. The court made this decision based on the Emergency Medical Treatment and Active Labor Act,[9] a decision made in spite of the medical knowledge that such an infant can never become a person and cannot survive. The child was kept alive for two and a half years with no hope of recovery and no chance of ever achieving anything remotely resembling human life. The emotional cost to the family and the financial costs to society were staggering. This case set the precedent for distortions in the interpretation of the PSDA that are far removed from its original intent. It is no longer a matter of a patient being able to refuse certain treatments, it now seems to mean that patients and families can demand *any* treatment, even if it is inappropriate, hopeless, and against the physician's recommendations.*

A Classic Example of Inappropriate Care in the Absence of an Advance Directive

The case of Helga Wanglie was similar to the Baby K case. She endured a protracted medicalized death awash in intense disagreement between physicians and family, negative emotions on all side, and costly legal entanglements. Mrs. Wanglie was an 86-year-old woman in a persistent vegetative state. She lingered in an Intensive Care Unit on a ventilator for over a year. Her husband wanted to continue care, despite the physicians' assertion that she would not benefit from further therapy. Mrs. Wanglie died of sepsis just days after a court found in favor of her husband.

---

*(To read more, see Appendix 3: The Baby K Case.)

Dr. Marcia Angell, former editor of the *New England Journal of Medicine*, weighing in on the Wanglie case, commented that on medical grounds, the definition of brain death should be extended to include those without a functional cerebral cortex (persistent vegetative state), but that the medical community had yet to adequately deal with this issue. Also, Dr. Angell agreed that patients and their families do not have the right to demand any therapy they choose; rather their authority is limited to refusing treatment or choosing between various beneficial treatments. But in this special case because of lack of clarity in the definition of death of those in a persistent vegetative state, the court made the correct decision to follow the wishes of the family. Thus, although this case was the reverse of the desire of the Quinlan and Cruzan families to withdraw therapy, it is consistent from a family value point of view with those cases since the medical community had/has yet to establish that a permanent vegetative death is equivalent to death.[10]

The Wanglie case again emphasizes the need for the medical community to address the equivalency of the persistent vegetative state, as defined as an irreversible loss of the cerebral cortex and death. Mrs. Wanglie had a protracted death with no chance of recovery. Her family had a death watch vigil for over one year that must have caused considerable emotional trauma. The medical team spent time and energy on a case they could not help while other ICU patients who could have benefited from care received less attention and were witnesses to this human tragedy. The medical profession, instead of organizing to deal with the persistent vegetative state and a real-time appropriate care review system, has instead become more confused as to their authority and that of the patient/family.

When there is no advance directive, misinterpretations of what constitutes acceptable care are common. The following case, paraphrased from a report by the *Kalamazoo Gazette*, in 2006,[11] is a classic example.

A Tragic Example of Judge Playing Doctor

A 97-year-old woman had a recent heart attack, failing kidneys, and progressive loss of mental activity. She was being sustained by a feeding tube, which resulted in frequent spillage of gastric contents into her lungs. This led to the need for a breathing tube to be placed down her windpipe, and a ventilator to help sustain her breathing. Because of infections, she was also treated with a series of potent anti-infectious agents.

Her attending physician in the ICU of a smaller community hospital asked the probate court to allow her "full code" status to be changed, her "breathing tube removed," and measures instituted to make her comfortable. He remarked that it was becoming more of a struggle for the hospital staff to walk in her room as her suffering escalated and her wishes were being neglected, perhaps ignored. The patient pushed away staff, writing, "I want tubes out, and I want to die, help me."

The newspaper reported that the patient was not married, had no children, and had outlived all of her friends. A court-appointed guardian directed her care and approved the physician's recommendation of a do not resuscitate (DNR) order. The judge refused the petition, stating a ruling by a previous state attorney general, now governor, that "Only adults of sound mind may execute a Do Not Resuscitate order, and may do so only on their own behalf. The legislature has not authorized a guardian to sign a DNR order on behalf of his or her ward."

The judge in this case felt that the doctor was overstepping his bounds in making the request.[12] He stated that a physician should not advocate to the court for the removal of apparatus being used to keep his or her patient alive, and that the physician's role should be to advise the family or guardian, and at most offer an opinion.

After approximately one month at the smaller hospital, her guardian had her transferred to a larger referral hospital, insisting that every possible measure be done regardless of her overall condition. At the referral hospital, she was transferred to the ICU the day after admission, was again intubated (breathing tube down her throat), placed on a respirator, and received various antibiotics. Because the court ruled that everything should be done to save her life, the hospital staff felt they were unable to follow her wishes and let her die.

She was discharged from the referral hospital to her nursing home but was returned to the larger hospital after only three hours. She was severely malnourished and had developed antibiotic-resistant bacteria in her respiratory and urinary tracts. She had severe dementia, fluid retention, and renal failure and was referred to another chronic care facility at the request of the guardian approximately one and a half months after admission to the smaller hospital.

After one month in the new facility (two and a half months after initial admission) she had no awareness of her surroundings, still needed mechanical ventilation, and required a feeding tube and multiple antibiotics. The new physician caring for her also felt this was abuse of a dying woman, but his hands were tied because of the court's actions.

Although both medicine and law deal with judgment, medicine must consider not only the emotional and physical manifestations and potential consequences of a disease process but also how the disease process is affecting the overall health of that individual considering his or her age and any other illnesses. Judges do not examine patients; they are trained to interpret legal precedent, not to integrate the multiple factors that go into a medical decision. It is my impression that in our society every court case should be decided on its individual merits. Shouldn't a judge try to gather as many independent medical facts about a patient as possible from experts before rendering an opinion on that specific case? She or he would most certainly want the unique facts about an individual placed into evidence in a civil or criminal case. Why aren't these legal standards followed in end-of-life medical situations?

It is not always the courts and the families who insist on inappropriate care. Often fearing legal action, the general feeling among physicians and hospitals in the absence of an advance directive is that all possible therapies, regardless of merit or possible outcome, must be undertaken. Families are often baffled by it all and are thrust into an extended and unnecessary grieving process. In the end, though, physicians can say "we've done everything possible," and the hospitals have made money.

> *Is it strange, bizarre even, that our standard legal procedures and rules of evidence are not used in end-of-life cases taken before a judge?*

Inappropriate Use of CPR in the Absence of Advance Directives or DNR Orders

As I mentioned briefly in Chapter 1, routine CPR was introduced in hospitals at a time when the average patient age was lower than it is now. Today's patient population is older, and the numbers of elderly in our hospitals will continue to rise. Still CPR is performed in end-of-life situations unless there is an advance directive or DNR order in place, even if it is likely to be a futile effort.

Writing in the *New England Journal of Medicine*, L. J. Blackhall observes:

Too often CPR just happens, without inquiry into the patient's wishes or consideration of its chances of success. Both patient autonomy and physician responsibility are important factors in making decisions regarding CPR. In cases in which CPR has any potential for success, the principle of patient autonomy dictates the patient's right to choose or refuse such treatment. The issue of patient autonomy is irrelevant, however, when CPR has no potential benefit. Here, the physician's duty to provide responsible medical care precludes CPR, either as a routine process in the absence of a decision by a patient or as a response to a patient's misguided request for such treatment in the absence of adequate information. In such cases the physician should not offer CPR. Both physicians and patients must come to terms with the inability of medicine to postpone death indefinitely.[13]

The decision to perform CPR should be based on the overall condition of the patient, and like all other medical procedures, when indicated, it would be ordered with the consent of the patient/family. Thus, patients in an end-of-life situation would be spared the indignity of having a procedure that frequently breaks ribs, damages the larynx, and involves intracardiac injections with little chance of benefit.

Some hospitals do have policies regarding physicians writing DNR orders, even against family wishes. Still, there are many barriers to withholding CPR.[14]

1. Covering physicians may be unsure of the patient's or family's wishes and opt for doing CPR.

   2. Physicians may be unwilling to address these issues with patients and
      families they do not know and have not taken care of in the past.
   3. Physicians might choose to perform CPR rather than face the possibil-
      ity of a lawsuit.
   4. Families may feel they are deserting their loved one if they authorize a
      DNR order.
   5. The topic may have not been raised with the family, and the patient
      may not be able to make decisions.
   6. Many teaching hospitals will not allow house staff to decide if CPR can
      be bypassed and thus in off-hours and on weekends CPR takes place.
      This raises the concern that the act of doing CPR may become the
      default response to a critically ill patient rather than considering the
      potential futility of such heroic measures.

At Beth Israel hospital in Boston, 294 consecutive patients received CPR
after suffering a cardiac arrest. During the 18-month study, 44 percent responded,
but only 14 percent survived to
be discharged from the hospital.

Eliminating CPR in the most futile cases would save
approximately $13 billion a year.

Ten percent were still alive after
approximately one year. No patient with sepsis (with systemic
signs of infection) survived. There was a 95 percent mortality for patients who
were homebound, hypotensive, or had a diagnosis of renal failure, pneumonia, or
cancer, versus a 34 percent mortality for patients without these other complicating factors.[15] In another study, 89 patients with terminal cancer received CPR,
but none survived to leave the hospital. Thirty-three were revived, but ended up
in long, expensive admissions to ICUs. Only one of seventy-three patients
(1.4 percent) with sepsis who received CPR survived to leave the hospital.[16]

As you can imagine, the human emotional cost of this kind of often needless
action is enormous. But what of the financial cost? Using data from the Beth
Israel study cited earlier, I created Table 2.1 to calculate the cost of performing
CPR in the United States. As illustrated in the table, the cost includes all the
care following resuscitation when the end result is still inevitable death. The
figures are staggering.

Eliminating CPR in the most obvious end-of-life cases would in no way decrease the survival rate. Reducing the use of CPR by 50 percent, eliminating the
most futile cases, would increase the long-term survival rate to 20 percent. This
single step could save the American healthcare system approximately $13 billion
per year, allow our hospital-based physicians to spend more time on patients they
can help, and eliminate the suffering of patients who initially survive resuscitation,
only to spend days to weeks in an ICU before they die.

Escalating Use of ICUs

When patients do not have an advance directive, is it often assumed that they
want everything done that *can* be done, whether it may have any positive outcome
or not. More and more we are seeing patients at the end of their lives receiving

Table 2.1. Estimated Cost of In-Hospital Cardiopulmonary Resuscitation (Codes) per Year

196 Codes using CPR per year at one hospital (Beth Israel).[a]

Of these codes, 21 patients were alive a year later (10.5%).[b]

Estimated cost per code: $43,565.00[c]
> This cost includes not only the CPR but all of the care provided following resuscitation.

Approximately 1,512,500 people die in hospitals per year (60.5% of all U.S. deaths).[d]

605,000 of those deaths came after at least one resuscitation.[e]

Multiplying those deaths (605,000) by the estimated cost per code from the Beth Israel study ($43,565.00) yields the astounding figure of $26.3 billion as the estimated total cost of in-hospital codes per year.

[a] Bedell SE, Delbanco TL. Survival after cardiopulmonary resuscitation in the hospital. *N Engl J Med* 1983;309:569–576 (PMID 6877286).

[b] Ibid.

[c] Lee KH, Angus DC, Abramson NS. Cardiopulmonary resuscitation: what cost to cheat death? *Crit Care Med* 1996;24:2046–2052 (PMID 8968275).

[d] See www.nap.edu/readingroom/books/approaching/2html (accessed November 2006).

[e] Thel MC, O'Connor MD. Cardiopulmonary resuscitation: historical perspective to recent investigations. *Am Heart J* 1999;137:39–48 (PMID 9878935).

care in ICU, rather than being made comfortable with palliative care in a general hospital bed or in the care of hospice.

Fees for ICUs are significantly higher than regular hospital care.[17] Hospitals have been increasing their percentage of ICU beds while decreasing regular care beds.[18] Is this practice in the patient's and nation's best interest? Consider the following data.

A recent study took a look at why Medicare expenditures during the last year of life have not decreased, in spite of the increasing use of hospice.[19] Their sample of inpatients revealed:

- The cost increased about 60 percent, from $58 billion in 1985 to $90 billion in 1999.
- The proportion of patients with one or more ICU admissions increased by approximately 5 percent among those who died compared to approximately 2 percent among survivors.
- There was a 10 percent increase in procedures in patients who died versus a 3 percent increase among survivors.
- In 1999, 50 percent of feeding tubes, 60 percent of intubations/tracheotomies, and 75 percent of CPR were in hospitalized patients who died during that hospitalization.
- Although the proportion of Medicare patients dying in a hospital decreased, those admitted to the ICU during their terminal admission increased, as did the proportion of patients having additional intensive care procedures.

- One-fifth of these patients received mechanical ventilation, even though death was imminent.
- Per capita hospital expenditures, ICU admissions, and intensive care procedures were higher among patients who died.

Another study reviewed 552,157 deaths from six states in 1999.[20] Thirty-eight percent were in-hospital and 22 percent occurred after ICU admissions. It was projected that nationwide, approximately 540,000 people die after ICU admission each year in the United States. The average length of stay was approximately 13 days, with a cost of about $24,500/patient. It is estimated that 20 percent of Americans who die in the hospital do so in the ICU. Do the math!

> I asked fifteen ICU physicians from all over the country, "About how many of your ICU patients should be in hospice?" The answer was approximately one-third.

A 1995 study conducted on potentially ineffective care (PIC) in the ICU of a large teaching hospital concluded that if physicians would identify patients who would die in the hospital or shortly after discharge, then they could focus more on palliative care for those patients and eliminate enormous human and economic costs.[21] The study projected savings of between $1.8 million and $5 million per year for this one hospital only. Imagine the savings nationwide if there was a shift in policy regarding ICU admissions and treatment.

With critically ill patients, is it feasible to determine that death is days, weeks, or at most months away? For a seasoned physician who has developed judgment after careful examination and discussion, I would say it most certainly *is* possible to make this judgment in 85 to 90 percent of cases. In the remaining 10 to 15 percent, in time, usually in a week or two, the outcome becomes more obvious in all but a very few cases. However, the important question to ask is, can this patient benefit from advanced technological care, and if not, why isn't the patient in hospice being made as comfortable as possible?

I asked fifteen ICU physicians from all over the country, "About how many of your ICU patients should be in hospice?" The answer was approximately one-third. When physicians in training are asked about this problem, by far the most common response is, "We just do everything for everybody; we do not make judgment decisions."

A patient chart review study from a teaching hospital tested the hypothesis that patients dying in the hospital had informed discussions regarding palliative care before being admitted to the ICU.[22] There were 252 hospital deaths during the time of the study. One hundred sixty-five patients (65 percent) died in the ICU. There was no statistically significant difference between general floor and ICU patients with known terminal disease that would skew the findings.

- The less experienced house staff referred more of these dying patients to the ICU than seasoned physicians. None of the terminal patients transferred to the ICU had discussions about palliative or end-of-life care as an option. Of those who died in the general wards, 25 percent had such a discussion.

- Patients who were treated in the ICU had more invasive tests performed and were less likely to have adequate pain control or be given the option of hospice.
- Of the dying patients transferred to the ICU, the cost was about $33,000 versus $8,500 for those treated on the general wards.
- Patients who died in the ICU did not live longer than general ward patients, had inadequate pain relief, and were not offered the alternative of palliative care.

THE AMERICANS WITH DISABILITIES ACT (ADA)

The Americans with Disabilities Act of 1990 (ADA) is a wide-ranging civil rights law that prohibits, under certain circumstances, discrimination based on disability. It affords similar protections against discrimination to Americans with disabilities as the Civil Rights Act of 1964, which made it illegal to discriminate based on race, religion, sex, national origin, and other characteristics. Disability is defined as "a physical or mental impairment that substantially limits a major life activity." The determination of whether any particular condition is considered a disability is made on a case-by-case basis.[23]

With about 2,000 advocates for this law looking on while this bill was signed on the White House lawn, President George H. W. Bush said, "This Act is powerful in its simplicity. It will ensure that people with disabilities are given the basic guarantees for which they have worked so long and so hard—independence, freedom of choice, control of their lives, the opportunity to blend fully and equally into the rich mosaic of the American , mainstream."[24]

The office of Civil Rights, Department of Health and Human Services, published in June 2000 "Your Rights under the ADA." A paragraph about physical and mental impairments was included. Those covered by the law, include, among others, those with "visual, speech, and hearing impairments; mental retardation, emotional illness, and specific learning disabilities; cerebral palsy; epilepsy; muscular dystrophy; multiple sclerosis; orthopedic conditions; cancer; heart disease; diabetes; and contagious and noncontagious diseases such as tuberculosis and HIV disease (whether symptomatic or asymtomatic)."[25]

The ADA is certainly noble in its intent. However, there are gray areas that often lead to inappropriate end-of-life care. There is no mention, for example, of what's required when the patients with these diseases or conditions are at the end stage. There is no mention that patients in the terminal phase of a disease should receive excellent end-of-life care.

The unintended consequences of the ADA make it difficult for the medical system to provide only beneficial care tailored to the individual even at the end of life.[26] Diseases under the ADA are considered a disability regardless of whether they are in an advanced stage and patients are near death. Thus, if such patients develop another medical condition under the ADA, they are entitled to treatment as if the underlying condition was not present.

Here's an example. A disabled patient with advanced end-stage dementia is at risk of a cardiac arrhythmic death. If there is no advance directive prohibiting the procedure, or a family member does not object, an implanted cardioverter defibrillator will be put in place. The patient will undergo a protracted final phase of life, receiving many cardiac shocks until death eventually prevails. This is excruciating for the patient. It is also extremely expensive. It is estimated that an implantible defibrillator costs about $100,000 per patient per year.[27] Here's where the confusion of the ADA comes into play. In one of the trials funded by Medicare/Medicaid, "Patients were excluded from enrollment if they had . . . any condition other than cardiac disease that was associated with a high likelihood of death."[28] An editorial accompanying the trial data stated, "The ideal candidate is at high risk for death from arrhythmia, but not death from other causes."[29] But in reality, the reverse is often the case. Many patients are at the end of their lives as the result of other diseases or conditions, but may also have or develop arrhythmia as a coexisting condition. Even though the arrhythmia itself is not the cause of their impending death, they are receiving these devices under the ADA.

PROPOSALS FOR CHANGE

We can fix the problems just outlined.

Address the Unintended Consequences of the PSDA and the ADA

There is a reasonable clause left out of the PSDA and the ADA that must be added by Congress. The clause could read: "Every patient has the right to evidence-based care tailored to the individual, but the patient cannot choose care that is deemed nonbeneficial based on the preponderance of medical evidence and the overall condition of the patient. The patient has the right to refuse any or all appropriate care."

- For the PSDA, patients of sound mind and of legal age may refuse any or all therapy where the expected benefits significantly outweigh the possible complications.
- For the ADA, patients with disabilities should receive appropriate care when the expected benefits significantly outweigh the possible complications.

These amendments are not meant for cases in which the outcomes are not clear; these amendments are meant for cases in which there is no doubt that the chosen therapy will not be of benefit. The anticipated advantage from this congressional action would make it clear that medical science and knowledge is an important factor that must take priority in medical decisions.

Create a Timely Advance Directive
with Each Hospital Admission

As described earlier in this chapter, advance directives do not work because few people have them. In the cases where an advance directive is in place, it may have been created years before and be seriously out of date. More important, it is impossible to know what one's condition will be at some future time. Many options that are reasonable at one point in a person's life may not be reasonable at another. All patients deserve individual hands-on assessment of their care, especially if there are conflicts. Administrative data and computer information are adjuncts to individual hands-on attention.

I propose a new style of hospital admission form that would create directives that are timely and appropriate at each hospital admission (see Figure 2.1).

This form would meet several needs.

- It defines who represents the patient—either the patient him- or herself, or a designated person.
- The patient states that they agree that they have the right to evidence-based care, tailored to the individual, but cannot receive care that is deemed nonbeneficial by the medical experts caring for them. Beneficial actions are those actions taken that will improve overall survival without doing harm in such a way that will diminish physical function, integrity, and dignity.
- The patient has the right to refuse any or all appropriate care.
- The trained professionals that comprise the physician team are responsible for defining beneficial care, where the anticipated benefit to the patient significantly exceeds the risks. There is an appeal mechanism in the event of conflict.
- With each hospital admission, the decision to order CPR would be made and noted on the admission form. If not ordered on the form, CPR would not be performed. If CPR is ordered, the patient/family may wish to withhold certain aspects of CPR that would also be noted on the admitting form.
- The patient can state wishes about end-of-life care and choices about hospice and palliative care.

With the best intentions, Congress created these laws to help Americans deal with end-of-life issues and disabilities. However, seventeen years have passed since these two laws were enacted, and the unintended consequences have not yet been addressed. These suggested amendments to the PSDA and the ADA and a new style of hospital admitting form would go a long way toward addressing some of the inhumane and costly end-of-life issues.

Figure 2.1. Proposed Admission Form.

Patient Name _____

Med. Record # _____

D.O.B. _____

Date _____

Is Patient capable of decision making { Yes ( ) No ( ) }; if not who is responsible?_____

A patient has the right to evidence-based care tailored to the individual, but cannot receive care that has no value. The physician team is responsible for defining beneficial care, where the benefit to the patient significantly exceeds the risks. A committee (the appropriate care committee) is available within the hospital should conflict arise. The committee will render judgment within one working day.

Cardiopulmonary Resuscitation (CPR) is ordered on this patient

Yes ( )   **No ( )**

The patient/family has placed the following restrictions on CPR because of personal choice even though it is medically indicated. DO NOT DO THE FOLLOWING

( ) intubation   ( ) chest compression   ( ) resuscitation drugs   ( ) cardioversion

Other therapies this patient has chosen to refuse even though medically indicated are:

_____

_____

_____

_____

When thought to be in an end-of-life situation by the medical team, I want to receive palliative care and consider placement in hospice:

Yes ( )   **No ( )**

The appropriate care I want is:

_____

Physician Signature _____

Patient Signature _____

Witness Signature _____

Source: © Copyright 2007, Kenneth A. Fisher, M.D.

CHAPTER 3

Why We Need Appropriate Care Committees

All patients deserve individual hands-on assessment of their care, especially if there are conflicts. Administrative data and computer information are only accompaniments to individual hands-on attention. However, there are many factors at play that keep this from happening, and which have brought us to the place of "one-size-fits-all" end-of-life care.

- Procedural medicine pays more than thinking medicine.
- In the past forty years, large training centers have grown into vast enterprises that need huge amounts of money to keep the doors open. The availability of Medicare funds has, in part, fueled this growth.
- We are in the midst of a large hospital building boom that is going to require billions of dollars to fund.
- The public has become consumer-oriented in regard to medical care and frequently demands treatment that has no hope of success at the end of life.
- The legal system is ill equipped to deal with end-of-life medical decisions, but an aggressive tort system is always present in the background as hospitals and physicians make decisions about end-of-life care.

Hospital rating and value-added systems based on computer-generated information cannot evaluate the best strategy. Only physicians, who walk the corridors of our hospitals day in and day out and stand at the bedside, are able to assess if a particular therapy is appropriate for an individual patient.

FACTORS INFLUENCING THE NEED FOR APPROPRIATE CARE COMMITTEES

There are several factors influencing the need for appropriate care committees. Let's look at each in turn.

Intensive Care at the End of Life

In Chapter 2, I pointed out that hospitals have been increasing their numbers of Intensive Care Unit (ICU) beds while reducing the number of regular care beds. Is this because end-of-life patients today are much sicker and have a greater need for ICU care and procedures? Although the numbers of frail elderly in hospitals have increased, it is difficult to understand how patients at the end of their lives today are sicker than in the past. Being at the end of your life is as "sick" as you can get, and there comes a point in time when all the treatments and procedures in the doctor's medicine bag are not going to make any difference. Or is the answer, perhaps, that a stay in the ICU generates more income than regular hospital care?[1]

Patients and families could benefit from active palliative care and ethics consultation in the ICU. A randomized prospective controlled study in seven U.S. hospitals tested the premise that an ethics consultation in the ICU for patients who were unlikely to survive would improve care and shorten ICU stay.[2] Five hundred fifty-one patients were identified as being in the end-stage of life in which conflict arose between the physicians and patient/family regarding the discontinuation of aggressive, curative care. Two hundred seventy-eight of these patients/families were offered ethics consultations, and the remaining 273 continuing ICU care. Mortality was not significantly different in both groups. However, the group receiving ethics consultations had fewer ICU and hospital days and life-sustaining treatment. All parties reported that the ethics consultation was beneficial.

A 1995 study examined the relationship between resource use and two-year outcome in 402 patients.[3] From a patient's lack of response to therapy, the researchers coined the term potentially ineffective care (PIC) and examined the cost of this care. They recognized that medicine cannot change the rules of nature and that when death is imminent due to irreversible multi-organ failure, it is time to switch emphasis to palliative, from curative, care. Palliative care rarely involves invasive or aggressive use of technology and as a result is less costly and more humane. The authors of the study concluded that patients in the PIC category consumed a large portion of the resources devoted to critical care at an academic teaching hospital. They suggested a change in focus from assessment of the quality of critical care and risk-adjusted mortality to an assessment of ineffective care based on outcome and resource use and a patient's response to treatment over time.

The worst outcome for ICU patients is not death itself but rather an extended death process in which suffering has been prolonged by ineffectual care.

The same authors published a follow-up article in 1997.[4] They thought that the worst outcome for ICU patients is not death but rather an extended death process in which suffering has been prolonged by ineffectual care. They concluded that PIC is common in the Medicare population and that these patients consume a disproportionate amount of resources.

Many studies, as well as many physicians and medical ethicists, acknowledge the need to recognize and treat acute illness but not end-of-life states, and that physicians must develop better judgment as to which patients will not benefit from ICU care. It takes competent and experienced physicians to decide when it is proper to abandon aggressive curative therapy and switch to palliative care. It is appropriate that physicians should be offering only beneficial care when the chances of improvement far outweigh the risks of treatment and its potential adverse side effects.

Appropriate Care Committees could come into play when a physician's decision to place an end-of-life patient in the ICU is challenged, when families demand ICU care against the advice of the physician, or in those gray areas where there is disagreement among the treatment team as what might be appropriate for a particular patient.

Large Teaching Hospitals and Their Style of End-of-Life Care

A study was conducted on regional variation in cost for the last six months of life for three diagnoses—colon cancer, heart attack, and hip fracture.[5] The study revealed that the cost of care for patients dying in heavily populated areas with large teaching hospitals was 60 percent more than in less populated areas with smaller hospitals. However, the patients treated in the larger centers did not receive better quality of care, and in many cases had inferior outcomes.

There is no doubt that we need large teaching hospitals as a place of last resort, where the most difficult cases are sent for resolution. However, all hospitals also need senior physicians with proven judgment who can help decide which patients are candidates for curative care and which are candidates for thoughtful, compassionate palliative care. The research just mentioned demonstrates that this kind of thinking is not taking place at our large centers.

In many large teaching hospitals there seems to be a mentality to use every known modality or technology to keep the patient alive in spite of an underlying awareness that such efforts are of no value.

More often than not, there seems to be a mentality to use every known modality or technology to keep the patient alive in spite of an underlying awareness that such efforts are of no value. Appropriate Care Committees are an excellent vehicle for making treatment decisions that benefit the patient, and set a better example for young physicians in training about appropriate end-of-life care.

Long-Term Acute Care

Patients in long-term acute care facilities have an average length of stay greater than 25 days. The number of these facilities has been increasing over the last few years, and so have Medicare expenditures for treatment. It is expected that Medicare will spend $2.96 billion for these facilities in 2006.[6]

As in other areas of medicine, for the appropriate patient, there is the opportunity for excellent care. But for the end-of-life patient, or the family with unrealistic expectations, long-term acute care becomes a setting for a protracted death with great emotional cost to the family and great financial cost to our society. Many patients in long-term acute care require prolonged mechanical ventilation (recently defined as 21 days or more for at least 6 hours/day[7]), and many of those do not survive.[8] In this group of patients, those older than 74 years of age and those 64 years and older not functionally independent, had a 95 percent (84–99 percent) one-year mortality.[9] Appropriate care committees would also be helpful in selecting patients for long-term acute care who have a reasonable chance of recovery.

Misuse of Dialysis

Congress funded chronic dialysis in 1972 and mandated that a medical review board screen candidates for appropriateness. Because of inaction, this requirement was removed in Public Law 95-292, passed in 1978. So, the Institute of Medicine has sought, and the dialysis community attempted to respond with, guidelines for which the burdens of dialysis outweigh the benefits.[10] However, these guidelines seem to have a little something for everybody, and conflicts arise often.

Chronic dialysis now accounts for about 5 percent of the entire Medicare budget and is growing faster than the increase in Medicare itself. However, is it possible to select which patients will benefit from dialysis and for which patients it is merely an unnecessary medicalization of the dying process? Appropriate Care Committees could resolve these conflicts and questions.

Nursing Homes

Many patients in nursing homes are at the end of life. However, if an acute problem arises, these patients are frequently referred to an acute-care hospital, treated, and if they don't die in the hospital, they are taken back to the nursing home. This can happen several times over the course of weeks to months. This shuttling of patients back and forth between nursing home and hospital when the patient has no chance of survival (e.g., advanced Alzheimer's disease, metastatic cancer) is unfair to the patient and is certainly inappropriate care. The local Appropriate Care Committee would help identify these patients and, with the primary care physician, inform the family that the patient has reached the state where curative care should be abandoned and hospice with palliative care initiated. Once hospice and palliative care has been initiated, these patients can now die with dignity and respect. Most important, this approach would offer the patient better care, and secondarily would save millions if not billions of dollars spent on futile and inappropriate care.

Cancer Chemotherapy

Appropriate care committees would be very beneficial in delicate decisions about chemotherapy for cancer patients at the end of life. A study of 1996 data revealed that 22 percent of Medicare patients start a new chemotherapy regimen in the last month of life. Within two weeks of death, the total was 18.5 percent.[11] This was regardless of whether the cancer was considered responsive or unresponsive to chemotherapy. The study concluded, "More people are now starting chemotherapy regimens closer to death with unintended consequences of late hospice referral and escalating costs."

Is it proper for physicians to prescribe therapies, knowing they will not be beneficial? Or has the physician not made it clear to the patient that the treatment will probably not provide any benefit and given them the option to refuse that treatment?

The PSDA, Advance Directives, and Legal Dilemmas

Chapter 2 covered these issues and the attending problems in depth, and the conflicts that arise provide a stage where Appropriate Care Committees could really shine. Some hospitals have active ethics committees and do their best to settle these issues. The American Medical Association (AMA) has an accepted protocol (see Figure 3.1) that balances the family's needs with physician professionalism,[12] but it is rarely used.

Many hospitals have suffered with the legal setbacks when end-of-life cases end up in court. The unfortunate repercussions have been that many physicians do not exercise their judgment and no effective physician-based mechanism has been created to support doctors in these situations. Sometimes it is the physician or the hospital that takes the case to the courts, seeking support for medical decisions, and is rebuffed by the courts. Yet hospitals, physicians, and medical societies have been reluctant to create clear guidelines that will keep these cases out of the courts, thereby preventing anguish for all those involved. An Appropriate Care Committee of experienced physicians could work with the attending physicians to practice benevolent and cost-effective medicine, assisting in conflicts about end-of-life care that the present ethics committee system has been unable to do.

Figure 3.1. Fair Process for Considering Futility Cases.

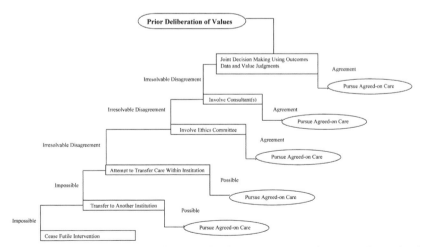

Source: Adapted from Medical futility in end-of-life care; report of the Council on Ethical and Judicial Affairs. JAMA 1999; 281: 937–941.

WHAT WOULD APPROPRIATE CARE COMMITTEES
LOOK LIKE AND WHAT WOULD THEY DO?

Currently, various insurance carriers, far from the hospital, review inappropriate care, and they use only administrative data to make decisions. The concept of a three-tiered (local, state, and national) Appropriate Care Committee system is a real-time proposal, creating a hands-on system of peers within the community with oversight by state and national committees for appeals and to avoid crony-ism. These committees, unlike insurance companies, would have no financial advantage in deciding that the patient now needs palliative care and hospice.

Facility-based local committees could tap program directors in medicine and surgery, senior physicians, and clergy, if they were available to serve. Subspecialty program directors could be members of the committee to provide input in their field of expertise. This team would be responsible for defining what constitutes beneficial and appropriate end-of-life care and be responsible for ensuring that evidence-based appropriate care is practiced throughout the facility. They would also weigh in when conflicts arise between physicians and patients/families, and when advance directives or DNR orders are challenged.

Some physicians might object to having Appropriate Care Committee over-sight that may limit their income. However, physicians have a primary responsi-bility to provide the most reasonable care for their patients and the wise use of resources for our society. If medical care con-tinues to be an ever-increasing share of gross domestic product, the alternative will be nonphysi-cian oversight that will create much greater limits on physician autonomy.

Local Appropriate Care Committees would be available to the physician who has decided that the patient can no longer be helped by procedures or attempts at curative care. When patients reach this stage procedures and technology are ill advised, they would benefit more with palliative care or hospice. But what if the patient or a family member doesn't agree? The committee would be available to assess the situation. If the committee agrees that the patient is now in an end-of-life process, then the beneficial and proper course is palliative care.

Representatives of the state-wide Appropriate Care Commit-tee would oversee the local committees and report findings to the full state committee. If approved by the state committee, inappropriate care charges would be withheld from future pay-ments to the physicians and the facility. The state committees would help ensure that the hospital committees are functional and would also review high-cost care such as ICU, dialysis, cardiac catheterization, and so on, for appropriateness. These committees would not question difficult borderline decisions, but rather obvious inappropriate care in patients who have no chance of significant benefit from a treatment or test.

Both local and state committee members would be appointed by the state medical societies and ratified by the national committee. Committee members would receive extra compensation for this responsibility, paid for by an indepen-dent consortium funded by all the insurance carriers, including Medicare and

Medicaid. Because they would be paid a flat stipend, financial considerations would not influence their decisions about appropriateness of care.

The national committee, along with its chair, could be appointed by the National Academy of Medicine. The national committee would oversee the system for fairness and resolve disputes. Setting up the Appropriate Care Committee system would likely require congressional action in order to give the committees the force of law, shield them from lawsuits, and provide uniform structure and function from state to state and among healthcare facilities.

What if a patient or a patient's family disagrees and wants to move to another facility that might provide the care they seek? They are free to do that now, and more often than not, are unable to find another facility willing to get involved in the controversy and take on the case. If Appropriate Care Committees become a reality in all healthcare facilities, then they would likely be met with the same decisions as the facility they are seeking to leave.

The establishment of such a system of oversight would also ensure that physicians-in-training experience a new culture of medicine that considers life and death as an inevitable continuum. Acceptance of this truth would not only encourage a model of more integrative care of patients and their families, it would also foster a stronger culture of compassion within healthcare institutions.

CHAPTER 4

The Three Most Typical End-of-Life Populations

It's not easy to say good-bye to loved ones at the end of their lives. It's even tougher sometimes to make the decision to end attempts at cure, move to palliative and comfort care, and begin the process of letting go. Perhaps it's a little easier with an older person who has become frail and who has lived a full life, but what about a terminal cancer patient who is still young? What about those patients who are in what has come to be known as the persistent vegetative state?

THE FRAIL ELDERLY

Frail elderly patients are by far the largest group facing end-of-life situations. As mentioned in previous chapters, the numbers will skyrocket as the baby boomers begin the trek into old age. Very often, these patients have a number of health issues, some of them chronic, some of them debilitating, and some that require specialized care. In many cases, that means long-term care, either at home or in a nursing home.

There are three general courses at the end of life for most frail elderly.[1]

Cancer

The first course is a short period of fast-growing, widely spreading cancer with a relatively rapid rate of decline. Death comes within months. Today's chemotherapeutic agents or radiation therapy may or may not affect the growth rate of the cancer, although we all hope for cure. If there is no cure, the amount of time a patient has left will depend on how much the cancer has spread, the location of the spreading tumor, the growth rate of the tumor, the age and overall health of the patient, and the response of the tumor to palliative surgery, radiation, or chemotherapy. Aggressive palliative treatment with chemotherapy, radiation, or surgery aims at alleviating symptoms to make the patient as comfortable and pain-free as possible. This means that the patient should receive maximum symptom control even if they choose to continue more aggressive treatment.

As the patient becomes more frail, when is it proper to forgo these more aggressive measures and institute only palliative care? The decision to continue treatment should depend on whether the expected benefit far exceeds the possible discomfort and organ damage. At some point, the patient will no longer benefit from any attempts at cancer-control therapy. The family, patient, and medical team must realize that cure is impossible, and all therapy must be directed toward keeping the patient as symptom-free as possible so they can still interact with family and others.

This type of care requires as much skill and attention as the previous phases of cancer therapy. These patients do not benefit from further hospitalizations at this stage in the disease process. There is more to be offered either by in-home hospice or in a dedicated hospice facility. Although it may be difficult for the family, the priority must be the patient, whose comfort and symptom control is paramount. There should be no attempt at cardiopulmonary resuscitation or ventilatory support in the event of respiratory failure.

Long-Term Deterioration of Organ Function

The second general course to the end of life in the frail elderly is a protracted time in which organ function slowly deteriorates. Patients with cirrhosis, heart failure, chronic obstructive pulmonary disease, kidney failure with dialysis, or other chronic organ dysfunction generally follow this course. Frequently there are bouts of worsening, followed by partial recovery, then another relapse, and yet another recovery. This can literally go on for years, depending other coexisting conditions such as diabetes or obesity.

When the patient has a recurrent bout of worsening condition, it is difficult *not* to hospitalize them and attempt to reverse the acute deteriorating event. One must ask the question, "Is the current illness another bout of deterioration from which the patent will recover, or is it the final event that will end the patient's life?" Things to consider might include patient frailty, the cause of the deterioration, whether the superimposed condition is reversible, and if there is progress in improving this problem over the course of several days.

After about a week, it is time for some tough questions. Is there improvement? Is everything being done to keep the patient as comfortable as possible? What are the chances for recovery? Have we reached the point where we should stop trying to overcome this deterioration in the patient's condition? If we are not yet at that point, what should we consider as we make a decision to switch to primarily palliative care in the future?

These are difficult situations, but is it fair to the patient to continue with attempts at curative therapy if there is no chance of recovery? Palliative care and hospice are the most realistic options. These patients and their families are in a particularly difficult situation. On the one hand, if there is any chance of recovery, the patient and the family want to continue curative care on the slim chance that patient might return to the previous state of health. On the other hand, if there is no chance of recovery, the humane option is palliative care and hospice.

Progressive Dementia

The third general course at the end of life occurs when patients have slow, progressive deterioration of cerebral function that over years causes the loss of the person, though bodily functions are maintained. Examples include multiple infarct dementia (many small strokes) and Alzheimer's disease. This is perhaps the most heartbreaking group of illnesses. Initially the patient appears well, but gradually, usually over many years, things deteriorate until the person you knew is gone.

As the disease progresses, patients become mute, unable to feed themselves, and completely bed bound. The stress on caregivers is tremendous, and eventually the families place theses patients in some form of chronic care facility. At this point the condition is irreversible, and nothing that can be done in the hospital can improve the basic situation. Therefore, these patients should not be hospitalized, and CPR should not be performed. At the appropriate time, they should be enrolled in hospice. Although it is extremely difficult for the families, it is, by far, the best option for the patients.

MEETING THE CHALLENGE OF A GROWING ELDERLY POPULATION

The Bloomberg School of Public Health hosts a Web site that is a thoughtful and scholarly approach to the serious issue of chronically ill people, a group that also includes the frail elderly.[2] Though there is a vast amount of information available on this Web site, I will focus on Chronic Conditions: Making the Case for Ongoing Care, funded by the Robert Wood Johnson Foundation.[3]

The facts are startling. Because of the success of many of our health research programs, there are now 125 million Americans living with chronic conditions; by 2020 the number is expected to reach over 150 million, most of them elderly. This success has led to another challenge to our nation's healthcare: the lack of an integrated system that meets the needs of the frail elderly who frequently have multiple chronic conditions. Our present system is geared for either acute hospital or nursing home care for many of these patients. What we do not have is adequate home care that would enable most of these patients to stay at home and still receive excellent medical care from appropriately trained medical personnel.

Our present financial model of health has encouraged a less integrated system than what will be needed to care for patients with multiple chronic diseases in a home setting. For example, physicians would have to be reimbursed for the total care of an individual with multiple chronic problems and not for individual visits, whether they are in the hospital, a nursing home, or at home. This would involve not paying for individual services but for the entire person as an integrated whole. This integrated system would have to include support services such as food, cleaning, and companion services as needed. Physicians would need to be trained in a different model than is now available at today's medical centers.

Today's physicians are not sufficiently trained in dealing with chronically ill patients, especially the frail elderly with multiple complicating conditions. I have heard, more times than I care to count, a patient referred to as "the broken hip in room 224," or "the knee replacement in 325." Patients should not be thought of as a heart, kidney, hip, or knee, but rather as an individual of physiological age, with various coexisting conditions, and a likelihood of one-, two-, or three-year survival given deliberate and appropriate healthcare. Physiological age is the health of the individual and that person's organs relative to what you would expect of the average individual at that age with that health. Some 90-year-olds have a physiological age of 70, while some 50-year-olds have a physiological age of 90, especially if they have a chronic disease such as kidney failure, cirrhosis, or advanced diabetes. Coexisting conditions (comorbidities) are health problems other than the problem for which the patient is seeking relief. An example is a person with Alzheimer's disease who has diabetes and a bleeding ulcer. The bleeding ulcer is the primary problem for which the patient is seeking relief, but the comorbidities are diabetes and Alzheimer's disease in its various state of progression.

> *Physiological age is the health of the individual and that person's organs relative to what you would expect of the average individual at that age with that health. Some 90-year-olds have a physiological age of 70, while some 50-year-olds have a physiological age of 90.*

Almost all patients who are frail and elderly have multiple health issues that need to be considered when developing a plan for treatment. All treatments have risks. The question to be answered is: Taking into consideration the overall health of the patient, does the expected benefit far outweigh the risks? When dealing with the frail elderly, frequently doing less is better.

The Art Buchwald case is an example of this.

Art Buchwald

Art Buchwald was born in 1925, and had been a Pulitzer Prize–winning humorist and columnist for the *Washington Post* for many years. He was elected to the American Academy and Institute of Arts and Letters in 1986. He was also the author of 30 books. Because of Diabetes Mellitus, he underwent a below-the-knee amputation in February 2006, and was told he needed chronic dialysis to stay alive. After a short period of time he decided to stop dialysis and enter hospice in Washington, D.C. He said that this was his last hurrah, and, " if you have to go, the way you go is a big deal." He made sure he had a living will to ensure that he was to receive only palliative care. To everyone's surprise, his kidney function improved as his impairment proved to not be fatal. He left hospice, summered in Martha's vineyard, Massachusetts, and completed his latest book, *Too*

Soon to Say Goodbye, after his five months spent in the hospice. He also included the eulogies written by his friends, family and colleagues.[4]

As a nephrologist (kidney specialist) who has seen many elderly frail patients receiving dialysis, I feel that Buchwald probably would not have lived longer if he was receiving regular dialysis, and his quality of life would have been far worse. Physicians and patients have to be constantly aware of the stresses created by most of our procedures and technologies, especially on the frail elderly. In many cases patients live longer with a higher quality of life, as Buchwald did by forgoing all but supportive care. Mr. Buchwald died at home in January 2007.[5]

Another enormous challenge is the nursing shortage, which is discussed in detail in Chapter 5. Most estimates project that over 1 million new nurses will be needed by 2010,[6] yet the number of U.S. graduating nursing candidates for certification fell by 25 percent between 1995 and 2002.[7] Approximately 75 percent of all American hospitals now have nursing vacancies.[8] The figures for nursing homes are just as troubling. How can we expect to deliver the kind care that our growing elderly population will need in the very near future without skilled nursing care?

TERMINAL CANCER PATIENTS

Many of the questions surrounding older people at the end of their lives also apply to terminal cancer patients. There comes a point in time where curative treatment is no longer effective, and to continue it would bring undue hardship on the patient and the family. Perhaps it is the physician who says there is no more to be done, or perhaps the patient simply doesn't want to face another round of chemo or radiation when the outcome is dismal.

As with most end-of-life cases, patients and their family members often want to know how long a person is expected to live. This is a hard question to answer. Factors such as where the cancer is located and whether the patient has other illnesses can affect what will happen. Although doctors may be able to make an estimate based on what they know about the patient, they might be hesitant to do so. Doctors may be concerned about over- or underestimating the patient's life span. They also might be fearful of instilling false hope or destroying a person's hope.[9] However, instead of focusing on a time frame, there are more relevant questions that need to be asked and answered. Would repeat hospitalization be of any benefit? Is continuing anticancer therapy of any value? Maybe now is the time to focus solely on symptom relief.

The patient's care will continue but is now focused on making the patient comfortable. The patient receives medications and treatments to control pain and other symptoms, such as constipation, nausea, and shortness of breath. Some patients remain at home during this time, while others enter a hospital or other facility. Either way, services are available to help patients and their families with the medical, psychological, and spiritual issues surrounding dying. A hospice or other palliative care facility is ideal.[10]

PATIENTS IN A PERSISTENT VEGETATIVE STATE

There are no consistent statistics for the number of patients in a persistent vegetative state in the United States. Depending on which study you read, it could range from 10, thousand to 40 thousand. One thing is for sure. These cases present some of the most challenging end-of-life questions for physicians, families, ethicists, and our society at large. The most recent prominent case that brought the persistent vegetative state to national attention was that of Terri Schiavo. This young Florida woman with severe brain damage ended up at the center of a heated national debate that drew commentary from every corner of the philosophical spectrum.

The National Institutes of Health published answers to the three most often asked questions regarding persistent vegetative state.[11]

What Is The Difference between Coma and Persistent Vegetative State?

A coma is a profound or deep state of unconsciousness. An individual in a state of coma is alive but unable to move or respond to his or her environment. Coma may occur as a complication of an underlying illness, or as a result of injuries, such as head trauma. A persistent vegetative state (commonly, but incorrectly, referred to as "brain-death") sometimes follows a coma. Individuals in such a state have lost their thinking abilities and awareness of their surroundings, but retain non-cognitive function and normal sleep patterns. Even though those in a persistent vegetative state lose their higher brain functions, other key functions such as breathing and circulation remain relatively intact. Spontaneous movements may occur, and the eyes may open in response to external stimuli. They may even occasionally grimace, cry, or laugh. Although individuals in a persistent vegetative state may appear somewhat normal, they do not speak and they are unable to respond to commands.

Patients in full coma usually require a respirator to breathe. People in a persistent vegetative state can breathe by themselves. People in a persistent vegetative state are also able to maintain an open airway. They can cough. All of this is controlled by the brain's nonthinking brain stem.

Is there any treatment?

Once an individual is out of immediate danger, the medical care team focuses on preventing infections and maintaining a healthy physical state. This will often include preventing pneumonia and bedsores and providing balanced nutrition. Physical therapy may also be used to prevent contractures (permanent muscular contractions) and deformities of the bones, joints, and muscles that would limit recovery for those who emerge from coma.

What is the prognosis?

The outcome for coma and persistent vegetative state depends on the cause, severity, and site of neurological damage. Individuals may emerge from coma with a combination of physical, intellectual, and psychological difficulties that need special attention. Recovery usually occurs gradually, with some acquiring more and more ability to respond. Some individuals never progress beyond very basic responses, but many recover full awareness. Individuals recovering from coma require close medical supervision. A coma rarely lasts more than 2 to 4 weeks. Some patients may regain a degree of awareness after persistent vegetative state. Others may remain in that state for years or even decades. The most common cause of death for someone in a persistent vegetative state is infection, such as pneumonia.

The persistent vegetative state from which there is no return involves loss of the cerebral cortex. You will remember from our working definition of death in Chapter 1 that the cerebral cortex is where the mind plans, reasons, remembers, and solves problems. It is the picture that comes to mind when the think of the "brain," and is the place where our alertness and humanness reside. The brain stem, at the base of the brain, carries out primitive functions, such as breathing, swallowing, respiring, and waking up and going to sleep. Terri Schiavo displayed these primitive behaviors, but her eyes were not focusing, her "brain" did not understand, and she could not interact with her environment. "With a persistent vegetative state the reticular activating system in the lower brain keeps sending signals, but nothing is there to receive them, no consciousness."[12]

The cerebral cortex is what we think of when we think of the brain. It is where our personhood resides. If it is irreparably damaged, the brain stem sends signals, but there's no consciousness there to receive them.

Often the brain stem continues to function, but the patient's eyes remain closed and he or she appears to be sleeping or dead. Sometimes, however, a person in a coma opens his eyes, yet remains in a deep coma. This is persistent vegetative state.

The most telling sign of brain status is an electroencephalogram (EEG). An alert undamaged brain emits rapid spikes of electrical activity. The persistent vegetative patient's waves are long, shallow and slow. Another test is the blood flow scan of the head that shows no blood flow to that part of the brain.

These cases present some very sticky questions when it comes to treatment, especially treatment of conditions that might be life threatening. When an EEG or blood flow scan or other test suggested by the American Academy of Neurology has shown no cerebral cortical activity, should treatment be withheld and the patient allowed to die naturally, or should treatment be delivered with the possibility of that patient recovering and continuing for years in the persistent vegetative state? As long as the working definition of brain death does not include irrevocable loss of the cerebral cortex, these dilemmas will persist.

DOCTOR/PATIENT/FAMILY COMMUNICATION IS CRUCIAL

Many respondents to my survey cited poor communication from their doctors when family members were at the end of their lives. Many studies have shown that patient and family dissatisfaction is often rooted in poor communication. Research over the past 20 years has shown that effective physician-patient communication is related to patient satisfaction, physician satisfaction, compliance, and medical outcomes, and patient dissatisfaction with medical care and malpractice claims are often related to miscommunication between doctors and patients.

As you will see in upcoming chapters, Medicare has significantly changed the landscape of medical practice, both for primary care physicians and physicians with hospital-based practices. It is often difficult for doctors to take the time to fully explain all the aspects of your condition; what courses of treatment might be appropriate and why; what medications are indicated, how they work, and possible side effects; and what the future might hold. Yet this kind of thoughtful communication is essential for dying patients and their families.

Talking to patients and families about death is often not easy, and some physicians are not comfortable with it at all. However, it can avoid many of the end-of-life nightmares that many patients experience, it can answer questions about options for care such as hospice, and it can ultimately bring a sense of relief and peace for all concerned.

Suggestions for Physicians to Improve Communication

1. Identify those patients that may be nearing the end of their lives. They may be terminal cancer patients, or frail elderly patients who have been in and out of the hospital, or they may be patients with a chronic illness such as congestive heart failure who are experiencing more and more serious problems. Patients like these have a right to know what lies down the road, and just knowing what to expect can relieve a lot of anxiety and fear.

2. Talk with them about their concerns. Perhaps it is fear of pain or of being unable to care for themselves. Perhaps they are alone with no family support. You can begin the process of educating them about palliative care and hospice and about community-based support programs.

3. Talk to them about unexpected events they have experienced in the course of their disease. Perhaps they had an episode of breathing difficulty that was unanticipated. You can make plans to meet future events, and reassure both patient and family in the process.

4. Bring up the subject of advance directives, and who can speak for the patient if he can't speak for himself. An advance directive should be completed in the later stages of the disease process, not years before, so that it is recent and timely. Advance directives advise the medical community of what indicated procedures or technology the patient does not want, including their right to forgo palliative care and accept whatever nature has to offer.

5. Since most of us would be more comfortable at home, educate the patient and the family about services and programs that are available.

6. Discuss treatments and procedures that will benefit the patient, and bring quality of life at the end, not just treatment for treatment's sake so that everyone can say "we did everything we could."

Questions That Families Need to Ask

Research over the past 20 years has shown that effective physician-patient communication is related to patient satisfaction, physician satisfaction, compliance, and medical outcomes, and patient dissatisfaction with medical care and malpractice claims are often related to miscommunication between doctors and patients.

In the best of all possible worlds, families will also be present, or at least informed, about all the discussions between the patient and the physician. Within the confines of confidentiality, the more the family is involved, the easier it is to chart a smooth course. Here are some questions that families need to ask, especially if patients are unable to speak for themselves.

1. What are the chances the patient will leave the hospital alive and have an acceptable level of human function? Level of function may vary from patient to patient. Human function may be defined as an ability to communicate in some way, possess some mobility that enables at least minimal independence, and have an acceptable degree of cognitive function that reflects awareness of the world and self. These are all cerebral functions.
2. What about some of the grading systems that have been developed? What is the patient's score and what does that mean for survival?
3. As days pass, what progress is being made? Is the patient declining, improving, or staying the same? What is the trend? This trend should become obvious over the course of a few days to a week.
4. Is this an acute problem that has a better chance of improvement or a progressive chronic situation?
5. Is there permanent and complete loss of the cerebral cortex (blood flow scans)? With no cerebral cortical function there is no human activity such as thinking, purposeful movement, purposeful communication, and so on.
6. Does an acute-care facility have anything positive to offer, considering the overall condition of this patient?
7. Is it time for palliative care and hospice? Should there be a consultation with the palliative care team to determine if this would be appropriate? Is the patient undergoing suffering that will have no benefit?

WHEN THE END IS AT HAND

In the ideal world, doctors and patients and families would have talked over many of the issues mentioned earlier, and the transition from curative treatment would shift easily to comfort care. Let's pretend it *is* an ideal world, and take a look at what the course of end-of-life care might look like.

Symptom Control at the End of Life

Patient suffering should be at the absolute minimum no matter what the phase of their disease process. This concept does not apply just to patients with end-stage disease needing hospice, but to all patients regardless of the trajectory of their disease process.[13] The Medical College of Wisconsin, Froedtert Hospital (Milwaukee)has created excellent guidelines for clinical palliative care.[14] The following is a summary of those guidelines for use by families, patients, and their caregivers. Simply having this information may help make the final phase of a person's life as comfortable as possible and take away the mystery and confusion many feel in this situation.

Pain-Relieving Guidelines

When possible, it is best to use the oral route of administration for medicines to relieve pain. If palliative surgery is required, oral and rectal routes of pain medication should be tried before the intravenous route. A fentanyl patch can be used for severe pain but not postoperatively. Intramuscular administration of pain medications should be avoided. Choices of pain meds should follow the three-step approach developed by the World Health Organization.

- Mild pain—aspirin, Tylenol, Motrin, and so on.
- Moderate pain—Tylenol #3, and so on.
- Severe pain— strong opioids (e.g., morphine), plus other drugs if necessary to control pain. In cases of severe constant pain, use long-acting opioids for baseline relief plus short-acting opioids for breakthrough pain as needed. *Every patient deserves to be as pain-free as possible.* Multiple long-acting opioids and nonopioids at the same time should be avoided. Bowel regimens to avoid constipation must accompany opioids. Postoperative and patient-controlled pumps should be administered by experts in those areas.

Nonoral Nutrition: Feeding Tubes

Patients whose death is imminent, and those in the final stages of a progressive chronic illness, deserve to be able to enter this final phase of life in as much comfort as possible and with dignity and respect. Although it is sometimes comforting to the family, nonoral supplementation does not prevent aspiration pneumonia (food in the lungs), infection, skin breakdown, or patient suffering, nor does it prolong survival.[15] Alternatively, the patient should receive pain and symptom control, moistening of lips and mouth, changes in body position, and spiritual support. These are trying times for the family, and meeting their spiritual needs is as important as meeting the palliative care needs of the patient. It is helpful to families to know that excellent palliative care is as important to the patient in this phase of life as aggressive procedural care was in the past.

Terminal Sedation

The intent of terminal sedation is to relieve suffering when death is near and symptoms cannot be satisfactorily relieved in any other way. The aim is to relieve suffering, not to hasten death; thus, this is not euthanasia. The actual mechanics of this procedure are straightforward; the impact on the family requires care, attention, spiritual support, and explanation of each step in the process.

THE CONTROVERSY OVER FEEDING TUBES

We will now step out of our ideal world and come back to the reality of the overuse of feeding tubes in futile end-of-life cases. Is giving nutrition through a feeding tube inserted directed into the stomach beneficial for patients with advanced dementia? Or a frail elderly patient with no hope of survival? Or a comatose terminal cancer patient? Although commonly performed, a summary of many papers found that there is no advantage and actually a significant disadvantage of placing feeding tubes into these patients.[16]

A feeding tube does not keep regurgitated stomach contents or oral secretions from entering the airway. A feeding tube does not prolong survival, and mortality due to the procedure is substantial. There is no prevention or improvement of pressure sores (decubiti), and feeding tubes in and of themselves can lead to local and systemic infections. In 1995, 121,000 gastrostomy tubes (feeding tubes) were inserted in elderly patients, 30 percent of them in patients with advanced dementia.[17] In large part this is because families, and many physicians and nurses, believe patients should not "starve to death," or that they should not withhold sustenance. Often organ failure precludes the normal use of these nutrients, so nutrition does not improve. Aspiration pneumonia (gastric contents entering the windpipe) is common, complications ensue, and life may be shortened, rather than prolonged. The overriding reality is that failure to eat and swallow in patients at the end of their lives is a sign that the patient is now in the final stage of the disease process and death is imminent, regardless of a feeding tube or other intervention.

In this situation, feeding tubes do not enhance comfort, and in many cases restraints are needed to prevent the confused patient from pulling it out, adding to the isolation and discomfort of the patient. As feeding tubes in advanced dementia or end-stage disease offer little benefit

A feeding tube does not prolong survival, and mortality due to the procedure is substantial.

and often create an additional burden, religious organizations now support a policy of not using them in these sort of circumstances. It has become clear, in both clinical practice and the scientific literature, that the benefits do not exceed the burdens.

With the public notoriety surrounding the Terri Schiavo case, the concept of feeding tubes has again been brought to national attention. There is substantial

confusion and disagreement about the legalities and the various state requirements, regarding the withholding or withdrawal of feeding tubes.[18] If the benefits
outweigh the risks, which occurs in patients with esophageal damage, or clinical
situations in which the digestive and other systems are not impaired, then a feeding tube should be offered to the patient/family. The patient/family has the right
to refuse beneficial therapy and that refusal should be honored and must not interfere with the caring relationship. However, if the potential benefits do not
outweigh the potential risks, then it is inappropriate for the patient to undergo
the procedure, and it should not be proposed to the patient/family. The physician's obligation is to attempt good and knowingly avoid harm. If the family asks
for nonbeneficial care, this would be an excellent situation for an Appropriate
Care Committee to decide.

PALLIATIVE CARE IS NOT GIVING UP ON THE PATIENT

In fact, it is just the opposite. It is part of the continuum from symptomatic control throughout life during any illness that may include the most technological
care. However, in an end-of-life situation palliative care should become the major
focus of treatment. Depending on the situation, traditional care may also become
palliative. For example, a person in an end-of-life situation with metastatic colon
cancer (spread to other areas of the body) may develop a completely obstructed
bowel, in which case surgery would be necessary to relieve the obstruction. The
goal is not to cure the patient, but rather to relieve the extreme discomfort caused
by the obstruction. Palliative care is not a death sentence; it is care given during
the last phase of life that is tailored to the situation and requires skill and caring.

What Do We Need?

We need a system that cares for the whole patient in an integrated fashion, so
that when technology and hospitals no longer provide benefit, care is transferred
to the home. We need home care capability that can provide cleaning, cooking,
feeding—all the necessities of keeping patients in their own homes. That means
many more nurses, specially trained in the care of end-of-life patients, particularly the frail elderly, to keep them in a home setting, to supervise less trained
helpers, and to know when to call for physician support.

We need an adequate number of physicians trained in palliative care, who
encourage holistic home care for end-of-life patients, and who do not focus on
procedures. Physicians must be capable of explaining that CPR is inappropriate
in end-of-life situations, be experts in pain and symptom control, and integrate
spiritual support for the entire family in the overall health plan. Most of all, we
all need to understand that for people at the end of their lives, less aggressive care
is often better care, with far superior results.

CHAPTER 5

Hospitals, Escalating Costs, and End-of-Life Care

Hospitals are often the last stop for patients at the end of their lives. While it would be nice to envision a place of comfort and care, where the dying patient's needs were met with compassion, it is, unfortunately, more a dream than a reality. This chapter examines how hospitals have evolved over the years; looks at some of the factors that contribute to expensive, inappropriate end-of-life care; and offers a few suggestions that might shift the focus back to compassionate, thoughtful healing.

THE EVOLUTION OF HOSPITALS

Ancient History

Did you know that in ancient times, places of worship were also places that cared for the sick and dying? In ancient Egypt, Greece, and Rome, the concept of caring for the sick was intertwined with religious worship. The ancient Greek god of healing was Asclepius, while the Roman name was Aesculapius. A temple for Aesculapius was built on the Roman island of Tiber in 291 B.C.E.

The concept of a structure dedicated to the care of the sick that was not primarily a site of worship is ascribed to Sri Lanka when King Pandukabhaya had lying-in homes and hospitals built throughout the country in the 4th century B.C.E. Mihintale Hospital in Sri Lanka may be the world's oldest hospital. The Indian King Ashoka built 18 hospitals with physicians and nursing staff funded by the royal treasury around 230 B.C.E.

The first teaching hospital with students and supervising physicians was the Persian Empire hospital, the Academy of Gundishapur. It was the intellectual center of the Persian Sassanid empire and under Khusraw I (531–579 C.E.) became an eclectic faculty-oriented (rather than an apprentice model) medical teaching and hospital facility.[1] It was the forerunner of today's academic teaching centers.

With the adoption of Christianity and with the First Council of Nicaea in 325 C.E., the church began to provide care to the poor, widows, strangers, and the sick. A hospital was built in every cathedral town. In medieval Europe, this concept of religious obligation to provide medical care continued. Meanwhile, in the Islamic world in Bagdad, there were sophisticated hospitals employing up to 25 physicians with specialty wards.

Early Modern and Modern Era

By 1500 to 1600, hundreds of hospitals in Europe became secular, introducing the concept that caring for the sick may occupy the realm of science rather than being guided and determined by religious thought. In the 1700s, the modern hospital, with its focus on dealing only with medical problems and staffed with physicians and surgeons, came into existence. In 1724, Guy's Hospital was founded, and in the Americas, Pennsylvania General Hospital was founded in 1751 with inspiration from Benjamin Franklin. He used two arguments in support of it: (1) remove insane people from the streets and (2) provide a place for workmen to regain strength to contribute productive labor.[2]

Modern Hospital Growth in Michigan

The development of hospitals in Michigan reflects the American frontier culture in the early to mid-19th century and after the Civil War. However, the evolution of the hospital industry in Michigan is fairly typical of hospitals throughout the United States.[3] They began as places primarily offering compassion and healing, and, as medical science progressed, they now focus primarily on technology and drugs.

Many of these institutions evolved from a primary religious entity into facilities that served the needs of a community in the midst of a healthcare crisis. Events like plagues or wars resulted in complex social, economic, and medical restructuring resulting in the birth of facilities designed to address these special needs. During the Detroit cholera epidemic of June 1834, Holy Trinity Church was converted to a hospital, and young women of the congregation acted as nurses. After the epidemic, the building returned to being a church.

St. Mary's, a 150-bed Michigan hospital, was built in 1850 with a gift from a private donor. Caring for the sick and dying became not only the domain of the religious community but a target for philanthropy, not only as charity but to further the understanding of disease. Government also began to play a role in the formation of institutions of healthcare. Wayne County, Michigan, paid for the care of some of the patients, and St. Mary's eventually became a hospital for wounded soldiers during the Civil War. Other hospitals had similar beginnings in the pre–Civil War era, and many served the government during wartime.

As commercial wealth increased at the beginning of the 20th century, there was a lot more money to donate to new hospital building funds. This new wealth laid the groundwork for hospitals as we know them today. Many of these newer hospitals created dedicated units for research and treatment of specific diseases such as cancer. Medicine was moving rapidly into the mainstream of society where it could enhance its service to the community, as well as increase its visibility to potential donors, researchers and universities. During World War I and its aftermath, tens of thousands of wounded Michiganders returned home, and the captains of industry, including Henry Ford, contributed large sums of money to create state-of-the-art hospitals.

At the University of Michigan, a university-owned 20-bed hospital was opened in 1869 and expanded in 1875. A new hospital was built in 1891, and in 1900, it was recognized as the largest teaching hospital in the United States. A children's wing was added in 1903.

The state of Michigan funded a multimillion-dollar hospital on the campus of the University of Michigan that was completed in August 1925. It grew rapidly.

- In 1939, a neuropsychiatric facility was opened.
- In 1950 the Women's Hospital was completed.
- In 1955 the Child and Adolescent Psychiatric Hospital opened.
- In 1969 C. S. Mott Children's Hospital, a separate children's hospital to replace the children's wing built in 1903, was dedicated.
- In 1972 a neonatal intensive care facility was added to the children's hospital.
- In 1976 an eye center was dedicated.
- In 1986 a new university hospital was built to replace the 1891 facility, and was expanded in 1990.
- In 1997 a new cancer and geriatric building was opened.
- In 2003, building began for a cardiovascular center, to be completed in 2007.
- In 2006, East Ann Arbor Surgery and Medical Procedures Center, the Rachel Upjohn Building, and a biomedical science research building were built.

This medical center is typical of the larger medical centers in the United States and represents a tremendous investment by a society that believes in doing whatever possible to relieve human suffering and extend life. But the capital investments and the facilities are so large that in many cases, good "old-fashioned" medical practice has been lost. The University of Michigan receives capital funding from private and state sources, and is the major referral medical center for the state of Michigan. Much of that referral is for highly technological care. Who knows just how much of that care is inappropriate? But as some studies suggest, the bigger the medical center, the more expensive end-of-life care sometimes is with no benefit and often with negative results.[4]

The Hospital Building Boom Goes On

We are in the midst of the largest hospital construction program in the history of the United States. The industry has spent $100 billion in the past five years, one and a half times more than the previous five-year period. This construction boom will increase the use of high-tech medicine and add to rising healthcare costs.[5] This construction is, in large part, taking place in newer, wealthier areas, featuring hotel-like amenities and expensive procedural medicine. Hospital bottom lines have improved, and with a decrease in the total number of beds nationwide, the occupancy rate is now higher. These factors, along with low borrowing costs, have made capital available for the building boom.

Hospitals are building and expanding to compete for patients that will use high-profit technology such as Intensive Care Units, cardiac angiography and stents, orthopedic procedures, and neonatal care, while putting less emphasis on primary and nonprocedural care. This trend also puts greater financial stress on inner city hospitals as they struggle with a different and less lucrative payer mix (more no-pay and Medicaid patients). Other factors fueling the building of new facilities include:

1. Areas of population growth.
2. Replacement of old facilities built in the 1950s as a result of the Hill-Burton Act.
3. Newer concepts in infection control and housing new technology for operating and procedure rooms.[6]
4. Consumer demand for privacy.
5. Anticipated needs of the aging Baby Boomer population.
6. Increased building of specialty facilities.
7. Rivalries between hospitals looking to outdo each other, creating a kind of "medical arms race."[7]

Hospital administrators defend all this new building as replacement of older facilities and adaptations to accommodate newer technologies. But mostly the financing depends on the anticipated income from high-tech procedural care, and quite a bit of this procedural care is performed on patients in end-of-life situations. No wonder that 27 percent of Medicare's annual expense of $327 billion, or $88 billion, is spent in the final year of an American's life.[8]

Medicare spends more than one-fourth of its annual budget on patients in the final year of life. That translates into about $88 billion a year. Much of that price tag is from unnecessary high-tech, high-dollar procedural care, as well as the financing of hospital building projects.

Academic medical centers are not left out of this building boom.[9] The Southwestern Campus of the University of Texas has a building plan to spend increments of $1.2 billion over the next decade. The University of Illinois at Chicago recently announced a $427 million hospital project along with four other academic medical centers in the Chicago area, slated to spend $3 billion on hospital expansion.

The vice president for healthcare at Turner Construction Company, the country's largest builder of healthcare facilities, said in 2004, "It's the strongest hospital construction market I have ever seen, and I've been in the business for about 40 years. I wake up and I kiss the floor every morning."[10]

HIGH-TECH MEDICINE AND ESCALATING COSTS

Several forces combined to give birth to our present style of highly technological, procedure-based acute hospital care.

Insurance

In 1929, Justin Ford Kimbell, vice president of Baylor University, developed a health plan for teachers that provided 21 days of hospital care for $6 per year. This was the beginning of Blue Cross/Blue Shield.[11] As Blue Cross/Blue Shield was able remain viable by insuring groups and not just individuals, the commercial hospital insurance business grew and prospered. With the advent of World War II, Congress enacted the 1942 Stabilization Act, limiting wage increases, but allowed companies to offer benefits such as employee health insurance plans.[12]

The next big influx of money came in 1965 with the passage of Medicare and Medicaid, to cover those 65 years and older, and the poor. Medicare expenditures consume an increasing fraction of the federal budget with care at the end-of-life a major component of that cost.[13] End-of-life costs also are a major part of Medicaid expenditures as Medicaid is a major payer for care in nursing homes.[14]

Before long there were other insurance programs, governmental programs, such as the Veterans Administration, Indian Affairs, military (active duty and retirees), and prisons. These all became new sources of funding for equipment, and reimbursement for costly procedures. A former head of the Center for Medicare and Medicaid Services has said, "Medicare has been turned from a program that provides a legal entitlement to beneficiaries to one that provides a de facto political entitlement to providers."[15]

Development of New Technologies and Medical Devices

Pharmaceutical and biotech companies have developed new biological agents for the treatment of cancer and other diseases. The medical appliance industry has developed cardiac and orthopedic devices. These represent the technological style of medicine that has become the expected and highly sought after standard of modern healthcare. Due to heightened demand and availability, newer devices and procedures are frequently used in situations beyond the range of their original descriptions, which were based on sound medical research and peer-reviewed studies. An example is the use of angiographically inserted stents (metal mesh-like devices with or without embedded drugs) for stable angina (chest pain of cardiac origin).

Stents often provide no more benefit than prescribed drugs, and billions of dollars are added to the healthcare morass when they are used inappropriately. They may not benefit the patient, but they are quite financially lucrative for the manufacturers, physicians, and hospitals.[16]*

---

*(To read more, see Appendix 4: In Support of Appropriate Care Committees, article titled "Cardiologists Get Wake-up Call on Stents.")

Financially successful hospitals are the ones continuously expanding their services. If someone will pay for a service, then the hospital will offer it. In the

> *In many ways, hospitals have gone from being spiritual healing centers to being costly high-tech centers. These need not be mutually exclusive if technology is used wisely and appropriately.*

era of subspecialty medicine, as new procedures and technologies become available and insurers agree to reimbursement, hospitals will provide the services. It doesn't seem to matter if the service is appropriate for a particular patient, and at this point, there is no physician oversight, like Appropriate Care Committees, to determine if the newer technology is only being used in beneficial circumstances.

Administrative Costs

Administrative costs for U.S. hospitals are enormous and continue to climb. Comparing administrative costs for healthcare in the United States versus Canada is both eye-opening and controversial. For those proposing a single payer, national healthcare system, the figures are quite demonstrative.[17] Data from 1999 shows per capita administrative costs:

- For insurance companies in the United States, it was $259 versus $47 in Canada.
- For employers' costs to manage health benefits, $57 versus $8.
- Hospital administrative costs, $315 versus $103.
- Nursing homes, $62 versus $29.
- For physicians, $324 versus $107.
- For home care administration, $42 versus $113.
- Total administrative costs per capita in the United States was $1,059 versus $307 in Canada. That's over triple the amount of administrative costs in the American healthcare system versus those in Canada.
- These per capita costs in 1999 translated to $294.3 billion or 31 percent of the total costs for the American healthcare system against 16.7 percent in Canada.**

Administrative personnel accounted for 18.2 percent of the U.S. healthcare labor force in 1969. That number increased to 27.3 percent in 1999. These increased administrative costs may be attributed to the following reasons:

1. Higher overhead that is intrinsic to private insurers because of underwriting and marketing costs.
2. Multiple insurers mean different billing codes and systems. That makes the claims submission process complicated and costly.

**(To read more see Appendix 10: Comparing U.S. and Canadian Health Care Systems.)

3. The costs to providers to understand different coverages and co-pays.
4. The increasing use of complex accounting systems, adapted from the competitive business community.

The problem of excessive administrative costs could be addressed by simplifying billing systems and by creating a national electronic medical record system through a semi-private government chartered entity, like the Federal Reserve Bank, to centralize billing and recordkeeping. However, if we were to address administrative costs but not the excessive use of technology, especially in end-of-life situations, the savings accrued by changes in administrative structure would soon be consumed by the inappropriate use of medicine.

Physicians must take responsibility for delivering "value" in the use of medical resources since only physicians can determine what form of healthcare is of value to a particular patient at a particular time.[18] The mechanism for physicians to provide value in end-of-life situations is Appropriate Care Committees, senior physicians reviewing the appropriateness of care individualized to each case.

Specialty and Subspecialty Training Programs for Young Physicians

From the 1960s onward, there has been a dramatic increase in specialty and subspecialty advanced training programs for talented young physicians to learn how to use these newer drugs and appliances. Funding for these programs come mostly from Medicare, with much smaller contributions from some other insurers. Pharmaceutical companies and patient care fees are also sources of funding.

The downside to this new training is that specialty and subspecialty training requires the mastery of an ever-increasing knowledge base. There is the danger that physicians in training will lose the ability to assess the overall condition of the patient, and decide if a particular treatment or procedure will actually be of some benefit.

Throw into the mix all the advertising by drug companies, hospitals, and specialty hospitals that give the public the idea that there's a pill or a procedure to treat just about anything. It only follows that people come to expect more procedural and technological care. We seem to have developed the notion that we can conquer nature through technology. Many people also believe that we have all paid for these advances through taxes and wage deductions, and therefore each of us is entitled to the "advantages" of this style of medicine. Excellent results are certainly possible in many situations, but more often than not, they provide little benefit in end-of-life care.

HOSPITALS, PHYSICIAN PRACTICES, AND REIMBURSEMENT PRESSURES

Primary Care

Primary care practices are the entry point to medical care and are considered crucial to a successful hospital. In-patient and outpatient referrals to the hospital are necessary to keep the institution active and financially viable. In the early to mid-1990s, hospitals and corporations purchased many primary care physician practices. In the process, they transferred many higher-paying procedures, like blood tests, EKGs, X-rays, bone density tests, and physical therapy from the primary care practice into the hospital. Consequently, the primary care practices were left with few high-ticket billing items, so the practices did not do well. Many ended up declaring bankruptcy, and hospitals and corporations lost a great deal of money. "If you strip a practice of ancillary services you should not complain when it starts losing money."[19] This statement is critical to understanding one of the major problems in American medicine. Hospitals must protect their bottom line while at the same time provide uncompensated care. They do this by maximizing procedural volume. When you perform more procedures, you get paid more.

> *What can possibly be the rationale for increasing dialysis of an elderly patient in an obvious end-of-life situation from two to three times per week to every day? This has happened!*

The present situation is designed to serve the economic, professional, and political interests of physicians, hospitals, drug companies, and insurance companies, but not the health of our citizens. We need a system that cares for the uninsured, provides evidence-based value medicine, promotes the centrality of primary care, and deals with caring for the frail elderly with chronic disease and the need for many medicines.[20]

Although Medicare has tried to address this inequity between procedural and primary care medicine by introducing the Resource-Based Relative Value Scale (RBRVS), this tool has not succeeded in preventing the widening primary care, specialty, and procedural income gap.[21] Thus, without procedures in the office, the primary care physician is forced to see far too many patients per day in very short visits, which leads to growing disenchantment on the part of the patient and the physician. As an example, under RBRVS, the 2005 Medicare fee for a 25–30 minute office visit in Chicago was $89.64 for a complex patient with multiple health problems. A gastroenterologist performing a colonoscopy in a hospital outpatient unit would receive $226.63 for the same amount of time, and $422.90 if done in the physician's office, almost five times the reimbursement for the same amount of time.[22] It is easy to see how profoundly this affects judgments about the best use of medical resources.

Starting in the 1990s, the VA system went counter to the national trend and mandated a strong primary care–oriented system.[23] From 1994 to 1998, veterans receiving their healthcare from the VA increased by 500,000, but hospital bed use decreased by 55 percent. Though hospital use by the chronically ill decreased, clinic visits increased by 10 percent. Survival rates for these patients were unchanged, thus decreased hospitalization did not result in more deaths.

This same correlation can be found in the private sector. Medicare spending in Manhattan, New York City, is almost three times higher than in Portland, Oregon. There is no significant difference in population health. The differences lie in the different styles of medicine. Manhattan is more in-patient, procedure, and subspecialty oriented. Portland is more primary care oriented.[24] In Manhattan, Medicare patients spend significantly more time in the hospital. In end-of-life situations, they were three times more likely to spend a week or more in the ICU with many more visits from medical subspecialists.[25] Not only is expense greater in a high-intensity, high-tech medical care setting, but also quality of care can actually be worse.[26] This is wasteful, leads to greater patient dissatisfaction, and may be a cause for increased illness and death.[27]

Physician-Owned Specialty Hospitals

If procedures using new and high technology were not so much more lucrative than standard hospital care, would we see the attempt by specialists and subspecialists to build specialty hospitals? This is a manifestation of a skewed reimbursement system that favors procedures, specialists, and subspecialists over primary care and compassion.

The physicians operating specialty hospitals claim they save insurers money by being more efficient as their costs per patient are lower than similar procedures at a full-service hospital. Their costs are lower because their patients are in better overall health. In fact, many are so healthy they probably do not need the procedure at all. As there is no physician-based oversight like Appropriate Care Committees, there is nothing to protect the patients and our society against overuse of these facilities.[28]

A study published in the *Journal of the American Medical Association* points out four major issues of concern surrounding physician-owned specialty hospitals.[29]

- Patient selection (i.e., "cherry-picking" of healthier and wealthier patients by specialty hospitals).
- Quality of care in specialty and general hospitals.
- Impact of specialty hospitals on the financial health of general hospitals.
- Influence of specialty hospitals on utilization and healthcare costs.

Based on my own experience as a hospital physician, I believe specialty hospitals *do* hurt general hospitals financially for two reasons.

1. They attract or get referral patients who are insured or have the means to pay for treatment, so that revenue is lost to the general hospital which could perform the same service. General hospitals are thus left with a much higher percentage of Medicaid and nonpaying indigent patients.
2. Specialty hospitals generally perform procedures only—procedures that could also be performed in a general hospital. Losing the revenues from these procedures is a definite bite out of the general hospital budget.

Because of issues like those raised by the American Medical Association and others, controversy surrounding specialty hospitals became a real political hot potato. In the Medicare Modernization Act of 2003, Congress instructed the Centers for Medicare and Medicaid Services to prohibit physician-investor referrals to specialty hospitals for a period of 18 months, ending June 8, 2005, unless the hospitals were already under development as of November 18, 2003. Congress mandated that during the moratorium, the Medicare Payment Advisory Commission (MedPAC) and the Department of Health and Human Services (HHS) conduct separate studies, with MedPAC focusing on payment issues raised by specialty hospitals, and HHS focusing on such issues as referral patterns, quality of care, and impact on the provision of uncompensated care.

Both groups studied relatively small groups of specialty hospitals, and only those that had been in operation long enough to have enough substantial data to study. In some cases, the data submitted was incomplete, particularly in the area of physicians' financial investments in the hospitals, and physician compensation. However, both groups were able to make recommendations including the following.[30]

- Changes to the diagnostic-related group (DRG) payment systems for specialty hospitals that are based on estimated hospital costs rather than on reported charges.
- More oversight to insure that the facilities meet the criteria for being designated a "hospital." The studies suggest that some entities providing specialty care may concentrate primarily on outpatient care and thus may not qualify as hospitals. That could mean they would not qualify for Medicare reimbursement. To address these concerns, researchers plan to revisit the procedures by which applicant hospitals are examined to ensure compliance with relevant standards.
- Stricter reporting requirements that would require hospitals to report information on a periodic basis about investment and compensation relationships with physicians.
- Stepping up enforcement of the physician self-referral and anti-kickback laws. Specifically, CMS intends to more aggressively scrutinize the relationships between physician investment and compensation and patient referral patterns.
- Setting different payment rates for out-patient specialty hospital than for hospitals providing in-patient care.

Through a survey recently sent to 130 physician-owned specialty hospitals and 320 competitor hospitals, HHS obtained substantial data with respect to Medicaid and charity care patient populations and found that competitor (general) hospitals treat a significantly higher proportion of Medicaid patients and the uninsured. Specialty hospitals generally treated patients who were insured either through Medicare or private insurance. However, no recommendations were made on this issue.

Although there is no fundamental reason hospital care should differ, the current findings suggest that physician ownership of specialty hospitals may be problematic if such ownership increases the use of services for patients with marginal indications. As specialty hospitals evolve, vigilance will be needed to determine if benefits are being delivered as promised and if untoward effects on the delivery system are emerging. In the meantime, all hospitals will need to look carefully at specialty hospitals to see what, if any, lessons can be gleaned from their successes and failures.[31]

There are also specialty hospitals that care for patients in obvious end-of-life situations but instead pursue aggressive care. Ventilatory hospitals, for example, specialize in treating patients with chronic lung disease, such as emphysema, who require assistance breathing. There are situations in which patients are transferred from chronic ventilatory hospitals to ICUs where the attending physicians supervise care in both facilities. Many of these patients are elderly, have severe lung disease causing them to require a ventilator for more than six months, require dialysis, have severe skin breakdown, and develop serious bacterial blood infections. Except in extremely rare circumstances, these patients have no chance of recovery and undergo a great deal of suffering before they die. By all rights, these patients should probably be under hospice care, but the ICU physicians frequently have the family decide whether to institute hospice or continue aggressive care with very little guidance or explanation of alternatives by the physician. Understandably many families are reluctant to make that decision. The financial benefit to the physicians and the institutions involved is considerable and without Appropriate Care Committees to oversee these cases, this happens repeatedly throughout the United States.

Physicians lobby Congress to allow specialty hospitals because Congress controls the funding for Medicare that will pay for the care in these hospitals. And physicians are not the only ones to lobby Congress. Companies that manufacture the equipment, devices, and drugs used by specialty hospitals stand to make billions of dollars in sales to these facilities, so it behooves them to lobby Congress to put up the funding for Medicare to cover them once they have been approved for use. Well-insured middle- and upper-class users of these facilities who honestly believe they are the recipients of something special, physicians who are more than willing to provide these expensive services, and lobbyists hawking their clients' equipment all result in a push for more specialty hospitals.

THE NURSING SHORTAGE

It is impossible to talk about the state of end-of-life care in hospitals without talking about the nursing shortage. Nurses are the backbone of hospital care. They are the ones who interact with patients on a daily basis. They monitor their progress and make note of reactions to medications or changes in condition, all to provide a more accurate picture of the patient for the physician who might only see patients briefly once a day during rounds. They can have a much more personal relationship with the patient, and the opportunity to learn more about their hopes and wishes about their care, especially near the end of their lives. They also have more opportunity to interact with the family during visiting hours. These are all important elements of good patient care, and especially important in end-of-life care.

Over the years, nurses have told me that the growing shortage is making it harder and harder for them to forge these kinds of relationships. They have many more patients to tend, and they have less and less time to spend with them beyond their required duties. They say they are stressed, getting burned out, and very disappointed that they are not able to carry out the kinds of duties that inspired them to become nurses in the first place. These are just some of the reasons that nurses leave the profession.

Another major reason is the emotional strain of working with end-of-life patients receiving inappropriate care. A 2006 study that surveyed nurses attending a national continuing education course on end-of-life care found strong reactions among nurses witnessing futile care with dying patients.[32] The most common situation involved aggressive treatment which they felt prevented palliative care that might have been more appropriate. Issues surrounding code status (CPR), life support, and nutrition with cancer patients, elderly patients, and patients with dementia elicited very strong feelings that futile care was far from caring and compassionate, and that patient comfort was often overlooked.

The shortage of skilled nursing care is serious, and the problem is growing. According to a 2006 report by the American Hospital Association, U.S. hospitals need approximately 118,000 registered nurses (RNs) to fill vacant positions nationwide.[33] Projections made in 2005 by the U.S. Bureau of Labor Statistics show more than 1.2 million new and replacement nurses will be needed by 2014.[34] Table 5.1 shows the U.S. Department of Health and Human Resources assessment of future nursing needs.

The nursing workforce is also getting older. Factors contributing to the aging of the nurse population include the large number of baby boomers who entered the profession in the 1970s and 1980s, declining enrollment in nursing programs, retention difficulties, and a higher average age of new graduates from nursing programs.[35] Findings from the 2000 Sample Survey of Registered Nurses (Health Resources and Services Administration, 2001) indicate that between 1980 and 2000 the percentage of RNs under the age of 40 fell from approximately 53 percent to 32 percent. The General Accounting Office (GAO, 2001) estimates that by 2010, approximately 40 percent of the RN workforce will be age 50 or older.[36]

The primary cause of an aging RN workforce is the failure to attract young workers (especially women) into the profession. The changing age distribution of the population will make it more difficult to attract young workers into nursing in future years. The American Association of Colleges of Nursing reports that enrollments in entry-level baccalaureate programs in nursing have declined every year between 1995 and 2000. Enrollees to these programs have declined by 21 percent between 1995 and 2000, while graduates have declined by 16.5 percent. The GAO estimates that the ratio of working-age women (age 18 to 64) to the age 85 and older population will decline over time from approximately forty to one in 2000, to twenty-two to one in 2030, and to fifteen to one in 2040.[37] This means that patient loads could grow even higher, leaving even less time for more than perfunctory and absolutely necessary care.

In a 2001 survey of registered nurses, 7,300 licensed nurses were asked why they are not working in nursing anymore. Twenty-five percent of respondents

Table 5.1. Assessing the Adequacy of Future Nursing Supply

Comparing the baseline supply and demand projections suggests that the U.S. had a short-age of approximately 168,000 FTE RNs in 2003, implying that the current supply would have to increase by 9 percent to meet estimated demand. By 2020 the national shortage is projected to increase to more than 1 million FTE RNs if current trends continue, suggest-ing that only 64 percent of projected demand will be met. The supply and demand projec-tions most likely bound the range of the actual number of FTE RNs who will be employed over the projection horizon. As the nursing shortage becomes more severe, market and political forces will create pressures that will increase supply, decrease demand, or both. State-level shortages will vary substantially over time and across States. As the nurse shortage in any particular State becomes too severe, market forces will create financial incentives for nurses to migrate to States with more severe shortages.

Projected U.S. Full-Time Equivalent (FTE) RN Supply, Demand, and Shortages

	2000	2005	2010	2015	2020
Supply	1,890,700	1,942,500	1,941,200	1,886,100	1,808,000
Demand	2,001,500	2,161,300	2,347,000	2,569,800	2,824,900
Shortage	(110,800)	(218,800)	(405,800)	(683,700)	(1,016,900)
Supply ÷ Demand	94%	90%	83%	73%	64%
Demand Shortfall	6%	10%	17%	27%	36%

Excerpt from: *What is behind HRSA's projected supply, demand, and shortage of registered nursers?* Department of Health and Human Resources, September 2004. Full report online at ftp://ftp.hrsa.gov/bhpr/workforce/behindshortage.pdf.

said they found their current position more rewarding. Twenty percent cited bet-ter salaries in their current position, 20- percent reported better working hours in their current position, and 18 percent cited safety concerns with working in a healthcare en-vironment. If you apply these percentages to the approximately 136,000 licensed RNs in 2000 working in non-nursing posi-tions, the figures look something like this:

Job satisfaction among RNs was lowest in nursing homes and hospitals and highest in nursing education. Thus, of the approximately 2.2 million RNs employed in nursing in 2000, an estimated 672,000 were dissatisfied with their work.

- 34,000 would find their current position more rewarding professionally.
- 27,000 would cite better salaries in their current position.
- 27,000 would report more convenient work hours in their current posi-tion.
- 24,000 would cite personal safety concerns with working in a healthcare environment.

Job satisfaction among RNs was lowest in nursing homes and hospitals and highest in nursing education. Thus, of the approximately 2.2 million RNs employed in nursing in 2000, an estimated 672,000 were dissatisfied with their work.[38]

Part of the problem is that nursing education itself has changed drastically over the years. The changes began as the focus shifted from in-hospital training for nurses to training nurses in the university setting.[39] Professional education in a university setting has increased the prestige of nursing, especially in the eyes of nursing leaders. At the same time, this shift markedly decreased the opportunity for young people from moderate or low-income families to pursue nursing as a career. In exchange for room and board, young people from modest backgrounds had been able to work in hospitals, training to become registered nurses. If they wanted to, they could continue later with university studies and receive baccalaureate and master's degrees and assume leadership positions.

Hospitals have abandoned their two-year residential nursing training programs, even though they provided us with excellent nurse personnel. Because these programs met our nursing needs, we did not have to recruit nurses from overseas, often from poorer countries who now desperately need more nursing personnel themselves. At this time, because few young people seeking a university education choose nursing as a career, approximately 75 percent of all American hospitals now have nursing vacancies.[40] Other solutions might include the following.

1. Recruit more nurses into nursing schools. To meet projected growth in demand for RN services, the United States must graduate approximately 90 percent more nurses from U.S. nursing programs relative to the baseline graduate projections. This will require extensive expansion of two-year nursing training programs, to attract students from modest financial backgrounds who might not otherwise seek nursing degrees at the university level.

2. Change RN wages. If wages for nursing services increase relative to wages in alternative occupations, then, all else being equal, nursing becomes a more attractive career. In the short run, an increase in wages for nursing services would increase the RN supply by motivating

- Licensed RNs not practicing nursing to return to nursing.
- Part-time RNs to work more hours.
- RNs to delay retirement or come out of retirement.

Insurance carriers including Medicare and Medicaid will have to increase their reimbursement for regular hospital bed care. However, if Appropriate Care Committees are in place to prevent inappropriate ICU admissions and nonbeneficial use of expensive technology, the savings would more than offset these costs.

3. Changes in RN retirement patterns. The rate at which RNs permanently separate from the RN workforce varies by age and education level, with high rates of departure between age 62 and age 65 as nurses qualify for Social Security and

Medicare benefits. There would be less impact on the nursing workforce if each RN were to work an additional four years before retiring. Delays in average retirement age could occur as a result of:

- Government policies delaying eligibility for Social Security and Medicare.
- A healthier population able to remain longer in the workforce.
- Improvements to RN working conditions that increase the likelihood that nurses will remain active in the workforce.[41]

THE PLACE OF HOSPITALS IN END-OF-LIFE CARE

When it comes my time to die, it won't be in a hospital, unless it's because I've been brought to the emergency room after my parachute didn't open while skydiving, or I've just wrecked a Formula I race car at Le Mans, and am pretty much DOA. I am exaggerating here, of course, but the message is, like you, I want to die peacefully at home with my loved ones around me.

Throughout human history, hospitals have been important as we recognize the need to alleviate human suffering caused by trauma and disease. Americans now spend vast amounts of resources on healthcare as hospitals occupying a central place in our healthcare system. But are hospitals the right place to care for the frail and those in end-of-life situations? A better question to ask is, "Can a hospital, with its technology and procedures, significantly improve the health status of this particular patient?" If the answer is yes, than by all means use all the available hospital resources, and deal with the cost. However, if the answer is no, then alternative places of care, like supportive home care or hospice, are far superior.

Unfortunately, for patients and their families and our society, there is no available information at this time to determine the percentage of patients in acute care hospitals that are actually in end-of-life situations and would not benefit from technology and invasive procedures. Whatever the number, it is most likely significant and unfortunate. Those patients at the end of their lives would receive better care, be more comfortable, live longer, and have better family and spiritual support if they were in out-of-hospital palliative care.

Palliative Care Training for Hospital Staff

There is no doubt that there is an urgent need for improved end-of-life care in our nation's hospitals, and this need will grow right along with the rapid growth of our aging population and the millions of Americans that will be dying in hospital and intensive care settings. Training hospital staff in the use of palliative care and hospice principles to provide better end-of-life care has brought mixed results. A study by Bailey and colleagues found that symptom documentation, care plans, do not resuscitate orders, and narcotics for pain relief did increase. However, the percentage of patients who died in the ICU did not change, and the use of restraints increased, demonstrating the difficulty in changing established patterns of behavior.[42]

The first step in this process is to teach hospital staff skills in the clinical assessment that the patient is in an end-of-life situation.[43] Appropriate Care Committees could assist in this assessment and provide back-up for the medical team. If staff resistance to change is deep, the committee may have to exercise its power to withhold payment for inappropriate care. As soon as the assessment is made that the patient is in an end-of-life situation, the patient should be transferred out of the hospital to in-home hospice care or a free-standing hospice facility. In those hospitals that do have in-house palliative care, the patient could be transferred to that section. Transferring the patient out of the acute care setting also reduces the risk of on-call doctors who are not familiar with the case transferring the patient to the ICU, a particularly poor place for palliative care.[44]

> Only 25 percent of U.S. hospitals have patient care policies addressing end-of-life or palliative care.

Only 25 percent of U.S. hospitals have patient care policies addressing end-of-life or palliative care,[45] yet hospital-based palliative care can have a lasting effect even after the patient is discharged from the hospital. Of 292 patients having palliative consultations in a large university hospital, approximately 37 percent died in the hospital, 37 percent were discharged to die at home, 16.4 percent discharged to an in-patient hospice facility, and 12.6 percent discharged to nursing homes. Three-quarters of the patients did not have a diagnosis of cancer. Of the 183 patients who were discharged alive from the hospital, 58 died within six months, some were readmitted to the university hospital but only 9 (5 percent) died in the acute care hospital versus about 45 percent nationally.[46]

SUGGESTIONS TO IMPROVE END-OF-LIFE CARE IN HOSPITALS

Appropriate Care Committees

As discussed, oversight by an Appropriate Care Committee could eliminate many of the costly procedures that serve no benefit to patients at the end of their lives. The Appropriate Care Committee could also preside over disputes between patients, families, and physicians over treatment options. This could significantly reduce the abuse of the PSDA and resolve conflicts when there is no advance directive.

The New Hospital Admission Form

Hospitals should adopt the type of admission form I suggested in Chapter 2. It would be especially helpful in cases where there is no advance directive or impartial individual with medical power of attorney to make decisions for the patient. The Appropriate Care Committee would support the terms of the admission form.

Training in Palliative Care and Hospice

Beginning in medical schools and nursing schools, aspiring healthcare professionals can learn about palliative care, and hospice options for end-of-life patients.

Using the palliative education assessment tool for medical education (PEAT) that I mentioned in Chapter 1, an entire curriculum is available, though few schools have adopted it.

Continuing education programs should include palliative care and hospice training. At the very least, hospitals could present seminars and workshops to make staff aware of the options for use within the hospital and in the local community.

Medical science has progressed and hospitals and treatments have increased in complexity, with dramatically improved results. The challenges facing healthcare facilities today are huge. They must raise the capital to build and improve facilities, equip them with the latest technology, and then be reimbursed for services rendered. At the same time, they cannot lose sight of their original purpose—as compassionate healing centers that operate on the principle of providing the very best care for each individual patient. For patients at the end of their lives, comfort and support may be the best care of all.

CHAPTER 6

Nursing Homes

Nursing homes are a 20th -century phenomenon that came into full flower when Medicare and Medicaid were signed into law in the mid-1960s. They provide both short- and long-term care, including medical, nursing, social, and rehabilitative services. Nursing homes that receive Medicare/Medicaid funding are regulated by the federal government, but many states have additional regulations and licensing requirements.[1] This chapter will look at nursing homes in general, including funding mechanisms. Then it will describe better ways society can care for people who have come near to the end of their lives than housing them in nursing homes.

A BRIEF LOOK AT THE EVOLUTION OF NURSING HOMES

Early 1900s: The impoverished elderly and disabled were housed in state supported "poor farms" or "almshouses."[2] These facilities were poorly maintained because of state efforts to keep the numbers to a minimum. In response, various ethnic and religious groups built their own private facilities to meet these needs.

1935: President Franklin Roosevelt signed the Social Security Act into law on August 14, 1935. This law provided matching grants to the states for old age assistance (OAA) to retired workers, but the people living in publicly funded "poor farms" were not eligible for these federal funds. It was the stimulus for the creation of private old age homes.

1946: The Hill-Burton Act was passed to supply funding for much-needed new hospital construction that had not taken place for seventeen years after the Depression and World War II.

Early 1950s: The Social Security Act was amended to require states to inspect and license nursing homes. The ban on financial benefits to residents of publicly owned nursing homes was withdrawn, and health service providers were then paid with federal monies.

1954: The Hill-Burton Act was changed to include funding for nursing home construction along with new hospitals. This codified the transition of nursing homes from the welfare system to the healthcare system.

1960: Nursing home scandals involving noncompliance in staffing, nonconformance with building codes, financial fraud, and patient abuse came to the nation's attention.

1968: Congress passed the Moss Amendments to raise the standards for nursing homes.

April 1969: Due to run-away costs, Medicare funding was withdrawn from financial support of nursing homes via Intermediary Letter 371. This change in funding was difficult for the many thousands living in nursing homes.

1971: With significantly reduced funding, most nursing homes fell out of compliance with federal standards. The Miller Amendment was passed to create a new class of nursing home—the intermediate care facility—with lower-skilled nursing requirements, and thus lower costs.

1972: Public Law 92-603 was enacted to provide Medicaid funds for nursing homes on a "reasonable cost-related basis" which, for the first time, also helped initiate a nationwide basis for nursing home costs.

Mid-1970s: There were still more nursing home scandals due to financial fraud and poor patient care.

1981: Once again in response to concerns about run-away costs, the Boren Amendment was passed to ensure "reasonable and adequate" reimbursement rates to nursing home providers.

1987: Following an Institute of Medicine report, the Omnibus Reconciliation Act (OBRA) of 1987 created new federal regulations for nursing homes.

1990s: Federal funding was granted for subacute care for patients needing more nursing and physician care than was available in intermediate care nursing homes.

1997: The Boren Amendment was repealed after the Balanced Budget Act of 1997 decreased Medicare payments to nursing homes, causing large-scale bankruptcies.

What is apparent in this series of events is that there has been a continuing national awareness that decent care in nursing homes is a social responsibility. However the costs continually escalate beyond the initial estimates, leading to recurrent crises in funding. It is unknown to what extent of nursing home costs are due to inappropriate end-of-life care, but it is certainly a significant amount.

MEDICARE AND MEDICAID: THE DRIVING FORCES BEHIND NURSING HOMES

President Lyndon B. Johnson signed Medicare into law by on July 30, 1965, as amendments to the Social Security system.[3] Former President Harry S. Truman was given the first Medicare card. The Centers for Medicare and Medicaid Services (CMS) in the Department of Health and Human Services (HHS) administer both Medicare and the federal component of Medicaid. Medicare is run and funded solely by federal taxes, payroll taxes by way of the Federal Insurance Contributions Act (FICA), and the Self-Employment Contributions Act. Total Medicare spending in 2004 was $256.8 billion. To be eligible for most Medicare benefits, you must be age 65 or older, have worked for ten years in a Medicare-covered entity (or your spouse has), and be a citizen or permanent resident of the United States. Those under 65 years of age are eligible if disabled or have end-stage renal disease, though there are a few restrictions and a waiting period.

Benefits for Hospital and Nursing Home Coverage

Part A—To be covered, a hospital stay must be seventy hours long starting at midnight on the day of admission and not including the day of discharge. Nursing home coverage is provided for those patients with a problem diagnosed during the hospital stay related to the initial cause for hospitalization. Only skilled nursing homes are eligible and coverage is limited to 100 days. The patient is entitled to full coverage of the first 20 days of care. From the 21st through the 100th day, Medicare pays for all covered services except for a daily co-insurance (co-pay) amount; which is adjusted annually. For 2007, the co-insurance for days 21–100 is a 20 percent co-pay. This co-pay might come from other insurance the patient has taken out to cover this sort of thing, out of the patient's pocket if they have the means, or from Medicaid if the patient cannot pay. Some facilities require prequalification for Medicaid before accepting patients who will be Medicaid-dependent for the co-pay.

Part B—This is medical insurance for services not covered by part A (usually outpatient), physician, nurses, X-rays, some drugs, and a myriad of other services. Part B is optional and if a person chooses to enroll, it is funded through a withholding from monthly Social Security benefits.[4] Many people choose this option because private insurance to cover the same benefits is generally more expensive. There are Medigap plans sold by private insurance companies that cover the various out-of-pocket costs of part A and part B.

Part C—Medicare Advantage plans are a result of the Balanced Budget Act of 1997 and allow Medicare beneficiaries to receive their benefits via private insurance plans.

Part D—Prescription drug plans became effective January 1, 2006. Anyone covered by part A or B is eligible.

The Medicare payment system is through regional insurance companies that process over 1 billion claims per year. There is very limited physician review of what is being billed, because there is no appropriate care committee system in effect to oversee the validity and appropriateness of care or treatment of Medicare patients.

Medicare now accounts for 13 percent of the federal budget. Medicare and Medicaid spend about one-third of all healthcare dollars, including 60 percent of all nursing home costs, 47 percent of all hospital costs, and 27 percent of total physician costs. Medicare faces long-term insolvency unless corrective measures, like appropriate care committees, are instituted.

Medicaid, the largest provider of healthcare coverage for the poor, became law at the same time as Medicare.[5] Unlike Medicare, which is funded entirely by the federal government, Medicaid is funded jointly by federal and state governments with poorer states receiving more funds from the federal treasury. The number of people on Medicaid increases when the national and local economies are doing poorly, and decreases with the return of prosperity. In 2004, Medicaid covered about 42 million Americans; coverage included about 60 percent of nursing home costs and 37 percent of childbirths.

INTERESTING STATISTICS ABOUT NURSING HOMES

Here are some surprising facts about nursing homes.[6, 7]

1. The number of nursing homes in the United States is currently about 17,000.
2. These facilities care for approximately 1.6 million people.
3. The average occupancy is 88 percent; average size is 107 beds.
4. Ninety percent of the patients are 65 years or older; 50 percent are 85 years or older.
5. Average age of admission is 79 years old with a three-to-one female-to-male ratio (in large part because women outlive men).
6. The nursing home population decreased slightly from 5 percent to 4.5 percent for those 65 years or older from 1990–2000.
7. Of the five common activities of daily living—bathing, dressing, transferring (bed to chair to bathroom, etc.), toileting, and eating—the average nursing home resident requires help with 3.75.
8. Almost half of nursing home residents are demented (impaired cerebral cortical function, Alzheimer's disease, multi-infarct dementia, or other neurological degenerative diseases).
9. About 1/3 of all nursing home residents have symptoms of depression.
10. In 2000, 67 percent of nursing homes were for-profit, 26 percent not-for-profit, and 7 percent government owned.
11. Thirteen percent of nursing homes are hospital-based.
12. Fifty-two percent of for-profit nursing homes are part of large chains.
13. Staffing: On average, per nursing home there are 52 total staff, 35 certified nurse assistants, 11 licensed practical nurses, and 6 registered nurses
14. Financing sources include approximately 8 percent Medicare, 68 percent Medicaid, and 23 percent private pay.
15. Medicaid: there are 1,667,319 Medicaid residents, 400,122,716 Medicaid days, and an average of $85.05 per diem (daily) Medicaid payment for nursing home care.
16. Medicare: There are 1,113,237 Medicare days yearly, a 27-day average length of stay at an average cost of $234 per day.
17. As of 2000, data from three states found that 54 percent of nursing homes were below minimum staffing standards for nurses' aides and 31

percent below minimum standards for registered nurses. This high-lights the national nursing shortage.

18. There is a large projected shortfall of qualified registered nurses, licensed practical and vocational nurses, and nurse assistants. In home health, the projected needs above 2001 levels will increase about three-fold.

19. In 1996, it cost $38,906 per year for patients living in institutions such as nursing homes, while those living in the community cost $6,360 per year.

20. Analyzing Medicare expenses, 5 percent of patients with the highest expenditures incurred 37 percent of all Medicare healthcare costs.[8]

21. In-hospital total healthcare costs decreased four percentage points from 1992 through 1996 whereas skilled nursing facility and home healthcare increased four percentage points, from six to ten percent.

22. The economic value of unpaid family care giving is estimated to far exceed the paid costs of nursing home and home care services.[9]

TYPES OF NURSING HOMES[10, 11]

Skilled Nursing Care Facilities (SNFs)

These facilities provide 24-hour care via nursing supervision (registered or licensed vocational), either long- or short-term healthcare, and assistance and therapies for the needs of daily living. These facilities are for those patients who need care 24 hours/day for physical disabilities; they represent our third level of care. The first level is acute care hospitals, the second level, long-term acute care.

Skilled Nursing Facility for Severe Mental Disabilities (SNFSD)

These facilities provide 24-hour supervision, many with locked or secure areas for patients with severe mental disabilities, such as brain injuries, mental retardation, and uncontrollable psychosis.

Intermediate Care Facilities (ICFs)

These facilities provide eight hours of care per day with intermittent medical and nursing care, meeting dietary needs, and some activities. These facilities are for patients too ill or frail to live independently or in an assisted living arrangement. These patients usually have a relatively stable chronic health problem but need supervised medical care for only part of the day. This is what comes to mind for most of us when we think of a nursing home.

Custodial Care Facilities

These facilities provide monitoring and other housekeeping needs and are designed to keep the frail elderly in the community and at home as long as possible. As our society ages, this service becomes even more important. It will need more attention and refinement, as well as more funding.

Reasons for Care in Nursing Homes

Some of the major health reasons requiring nursing home care are:

1. Loss of function of our most complex organ, the cerebral cortex, through
   a. traumatic brain injury
   b. vascular diseases, such as atherosclerosis or vasculitis
   c. degenerative diseases, such as Alzheimer's disease
   d. genetic diseases
2. Various organ failures, such as heart failure, chronic obstructive pulmonary disease, hepatic failure, bowel diseases, and many others.
3. Bone problems, such as broken hips.
4. Excessive frailty from old age.

There is a growing awareness of the need to develop services apart from nursing homes that provide care tailored to each patient over and above assistance with daily life tasks. The goal is to keep people out of medical institutions where the costs become prohibitive, and the care is often impersonal. As our population ages, we will see these kinds of services grow. These newer services require only a minimum of medical supervision and include:

1. Community-based services, such as Meals on Wheels, adult protective services.
2. Home healthcare with visiting nurses and assistance with housekeeping chores.
3. In-law apartments.
4. Housing for aging and disabled individuals, a slightly higher level of care but not medically supervised.
5. Board and care homes, a variation of number 4.
6. Assisted living that provides apartment living in a protected environment.
7. Continuing-care retirement communities.

PATIENT POPULATIONS AND LENGTH OF STAY

Table 6.1 outlines discharge rates for both men and women, based on the length of time spent in the nursing home. There is no distinction between patients discharged because they either recovered or were transferred elsewhere, and patients who were "discharged" because they died.

Here's how I would analyze these data.

Group I patients, the largest percentage by far, are those patients staying less than one month for both genders, 41 percent for males and 43 percent for females. This group of patients is probably those who are discharged from the hospital as functioning people who need more time to recuperate from their illness and then proceed home. Many of the rest of Group I patients (in the nursing home for less

Table 6.1. Nursing Home Discharge Rates

Group I (Discharged 12 months)			Group II (Discharged 1–3 years)			Group III (Discharged 3–10+ years)		
	Males	Females		Males	Females		Males	Females
<1 month	41%	43%	1–2 yrs	9%	7%	3–5 yrs	2%	5%
1–3 mos	18%	22%	2–3 yrs	5%	2%	5–10 yrs	5%	6%
3–6 mos	11%	7%				>10 yrs	1%	3%
6–12 mos	8%	5%						

Adapted from information at www.elderweb.com/home/taxonomy/term/6370 (accessed March 12, 2007).

than a year) are more frail, but, excluding those who died, most probably were discharged into a less structured setting like assisted living.

Group II patients (in the nursing home for one to three years) probably were discharged because of death because they were too frail to be placed in a noninstitutional setting. The major question for these patients is not how long they will live, but rather, if they have an acute healthcare problem, would they benefit from admission to an acute care facility? Almost all these patients may have their lives prolonged by acute care, but their overall downhill course is irreversible, and palliative care at the nursing home, home, or other hospice setting would be more appropriate.

A More Common Case Than You Might Think

Mrs. K. was a 76-year-old woman with significant atherosclerotic disease exacerbated by heavy smoking and manifested as cerebral vascular disease with multiple-infarct dementia. She also had coronary artery disease with a history of two heart attacks associated with congestive heart failure, and peripheral arterial disease causing skin breakdown and ulcers on both lower legs. Because of her severe dementia, she no longer had motor activity, could not move, and had developed severe skin breakdown on her back side called decubitii, which often serve as a prime breeding ground for chronic, recurrent infections. Stool and urine had to be cleaned from her skin wounds daily. Although completely unaware of her surroundings, she had been hospitalized five times in the preceding year. Three of her admissions were due to pneumonia, caused twice by aspiration of throat contents into her lungs, and once by excessive fluid in her lungs secondary to her poor heart function. The other two admissions were due to bacteria in her blood (sepsis) caused by her skin ulcers. She had two children, both living a considerable distance away, who visited her infrequently. She had no advance directive. When her children were called about each acute illness in the nursing home, they opted for hospitalization and CPR if she suffered an event that would require resuscitation. During three of the five hospitalizations she was in the ICU for a total of fourteen days. During each admission the nursing staff had raised questions about the appropriateness of all this aggressive care, which was only causing suffering for this severely demented woman. The doctors and hospital executives told them that their hands were tied because of her children's wishes, and the fact that there was no advance directive. Twenty-four hours after being returned to the nursing home after the last hospital admission she suddenly died. No autopsy was performed, so the actual cause of death was unknown.

Group III patients represent a tragic and difficult problem. These patients most likely represent nearly 50 percent of nursing home patients—those with degenerating cerebral cortical function, but who can survive three to ten years or longer in a nursing home. They should not receive curative medical care with the goal of leaving institutional living. They are on a path toward death because their cerebral dysfunction will only continue to worsen. Except in unique circumstances that would lead to more comfort or pain control, they should not be admitted to an acute care facility, and they should not undergo CPR. What they *do* need is dignified, compassionate care in a less medicalized setting that could provide that care in a less costly manner.

So, all nursing home patients are not the same. Those recuperating from acute care who have the physical and mental capacity for independent or assisted living should receive any level of care it takes to make them well. Those who are frail and at the end of their lives should be made as comfortable as 21st century medicine can deliver, but should not be sent to acute care facilities when life-ending events such as pneumonia or urinary tract infections occur. Those who are in the later stages of degenerative brain disease will not benefit from medical care, but rather need compassionate comfort care that can last several years. They should not receive CPR when death occurs. This sort of ill-advised unsuccessful attempt at CPR reflects our inappropriate use of CPR in an end-of-life situation.

BABY BOOMERS, MEDICAID BUDGETS, AND FINANCING LONG-TERM CARE

As the proportion of elderly in our population increases (from 13 percent in 2000 to an expected 20 percent in 2030), the expenditures for long-term chronic care increase. Expenses for long-term care also increase as we live longer. In 1996 dollars, a person dying at age 65 spent $31,000 for acute and long-term care, while a person dying at age 90 spent $200,000 for acute and long-term care, with most of the increase spent on long-term care. As longevity increases, acute care expenditures increase at a reduced rate, but long-term care such as nursing homes increases at an accelerated rate.[12]

Medicaid funds 68 percent of nursing home care. It will require significantly more funding and changes in structure in order to fund the increasing need for nursing home care as our population ages. As it stands now, Medicaid is not positioned to meet these increasing financial demands.

The Medicaid program has grown tremendously since its inception in 1965/66. Enrollment increased from 4 million in 1966 to 47 million in 2002. Expenditures have increased from $400 million to $257 billion. Two-thirds of these expenditures were for the elderly and disabled.[13]

Here's where things get tricky with Medicaid reimbursements. When a Medicaid nursing home patient who is Medicare eligible is admitted to an acute care facility, Medicare is billed for the acute services. When the patient returns to the nursing home, Medicare only covers a limited period of time (20 days full pay, 80 days with co-pay). After that, Medicaid is again responsible for the expense. Because Medicare payments exceed those of Medicaid, there is a financial incentive to shuttle patients back and forth between nursing homes and acute care facilities to get around the Medicare time/payment limits. Because Medicaid pays less than the actual cost, nursing homes need the increased payments by Medicare to "keep the doors open." The result: Yet more potentially inappropriate care, especially for patients like Mrs. K., who are clearly at the end of their lives.

In 2001, Medicaid spending alone consumed 42 percent of the increase in state budgets. Growth in state and federal Medicaid spending in 2001 was approximately 14 percent. Decreasing state tax revenues and increased Medicaid spending caused budget gaps in 43 states totaling $36 billion in fiscal year 2002. States used a variety of temporary measures to fund this deficit, including drawing down on emergency funds; taking monies from highway, education, and other funds; tobacco settlement monies; decreasing Medicaid benefits; and increases in taxes, especially on cigarettes.[14]

A June 2006 report focused on the Medicaid funding shortfall for its nursing home population.[13] The average shortfall for the country was $13.10/day in 2006, which was a 45 percent increase from 1999 to 2006. The national total shortfall for allowable costs was $4.5 billion. States have been depending on federal matching of provider taxes to help meet their nursing home costs. These federal funds are to be decreased. Even as states promote home-based and other community-based services for those people who can still remain at home, the average nursing home patient is less independent, driving up nursing homes costs. Medicare cross-subsidization of Medicaid continues to be a major backup to Medicaid funding shortfalls; if federal budget constraints decrease this subsidization, the shortfall situation will worsen.

SUGGESTIONS FOR IMPROVING NURSING HOME END-OF-LIFE CARE

Naturally, I have some suggestions for improving care in nursing homes in end-of-life situations.

Appropriate Care Committees

The case of Mrs. K. is typical of tens (if not hundreds) of thousands occurring yearly in the United States. She was unaware of her surroundings, had no human interaction, could not participate in any activities of daily living, and, had she possessed awareness of her body or her mental faculties, would likely have suffered significant pain and indignity, with no hope of improvement. In other countries, and decades ago in the United States, this woman would have been allowed to die with her dignity intact. Her children were in a difficult situation. They could not see that their mother was terminally ill as they lived far away, and therefore did not have firsthand experience of her physical and cognitive status. Thus, when called with each life-threatening event and asked, "What should be done?", they opted for what they thought was the best care for their mother. In this case, there was no professional communication to the family about the most humane or appropriate care for their mother. It not only prolonged her suffering, but may have misled the family into false hope.

This is a common occurrence in hospitals and nursing homes, and is a direct result of misinterpretations of the Patient Self-Determination Act. Had an Appropriate Care Committee been overseeing patient care and reporting honestly to the family, Mrs. K.'s last days might have been very different.

Palliative Care and Hospice

Although more and more patients are dying in nursing homes, as of 1997, 70 percent of all nursing homes did not offer hospice. Studies found that many dying patients had excessive pain, and inadequate end-of-life care, pointing out that standards and rules are aimed at restorative and technologically oriented care rather than palliative care.[15] Obstacles to palliative care in nursing homes include a lack of recognition that a patient is at the end of life, and that acute hospital care is no longer appropriate, This may be compounded by a lack of communication between staff and family that the patient is in an end-of-life situation. The absence of such rudimentary communication may result in the absence of an agreement on a reasonable plan of care.[16]

An article published in the *Journal of Law, Medicine and Ethics* examines, according to its abstract:

> current health care policies and government practices that deter appropriate end-of-life care, focusing on the use of hospice services for dying nursing home patients. The authors conclude that hospice and nursing home regulations, reimbursement for hospice and nursing homes, and enforcement of the fraud and abuse rules collude to "chill" utilization of hospice by nursing homes and result in inadequate end-of-life care for many nursing home patients. They argue that these policies and practices have at their roots a number of questionable assumptions and call for a shift in existing paradigms affecting care to this group and a realigning of incentives among these various government policies to achieve consistent policy goals.[17]

Other factors found to inhibit good end-of-life care in nursing homes include crowded rooms that are noisy, lack of privacy, and inadequate staffing and supervision.[18] However, concerted efforts made to introduce palliative care and hospice to patients and families have been shown to significantly increase the use of these services.[19] But there are still many legal stumbling blocks to first-class hospice care in nursing homes.[20]

Besides appropriate care committees, we need to create a legal framework to provide hospice care in nursing homes to address this national problem.

We face many hurdles in promoting excellent nursing home care. We do not yet have appropriate care committees that can help determine what is the best care for each patient. The major task for an Appropriate Care Committee in a nursing home is to realistically evaluate each patient. If the patient is recuperating from an acute event and when healed would be able to live independently, even with assistance, then every effort should be made to achieve that goal. In the classification in this chapter, this would be Group I.

If, on the other hand, the patient is in an end-of-life situation, palliative care and hospice are appropriate—in the nursing home, at home if possible, or in a dedicated hospice facility. These patients would be in Group II as defined in this chapter.

Patients who are losing their cerebral cortical function are increasing as our population ages. They slowly worsen till death, needing dignified chronic palliative care knowing that in the latter stages they cannot return to any form of independent living. Except for palliative reasons, they should not enter an acute care facility, and they should not be resuscitated when dying. This is Group III, as discussed in this chapter.

There are many community options being developed that need nurturing so that patients can remain out of institutions. It is far superior care for the patient, and it will conserve vital resources. Plans have been suggested that would shift much of the state responsibility for long-term care to the federal government.[21] Although this plan would help sustain Medicaid at the state level, it would put an added financial burden on Medicare. However, once Appropriate Care Committees were functioning within our medical systems, Medicare savings would be available to help support Medicaid.

CHAPTER 7

Palliative Care and Hospice

Palliative: Adjective; a Middle English adaptation of the Latin palliates, meaning to cloak, hide, or conceal, evolved over the years to apply to refer to reducing the symptoms of disease. The modern definition of palliative care refers to any care that relieves symptoms, whether or not curative care is also being attempted.

Before World War II and the advent of modern scientific- and technology-based medicine, what we now call palliative medicine *was* medicine. Physicians were experts in symptom control and grief counseling. This was the role of physicians in that time.

As money began to pour into medical research, scientific knowledge grew, and specialization and subspecialization became the new paradigms of medicine. Doctors were able to go beyond controlling infectious diseases to eradicating them altogether. Studies and research cast new light on genetics, molecular biology, cell biology, pathophysiology, and other mechanisms of disease. Revolutionary insights emerged from a deeper understanding of biology such as the structure of DNA. We gained new abilities to tinker around with protein structures in ways that profoundly altered pharmacology and our ability to treat diseases. As relief from the ravages of disease moved from being only a vision to being a day-to-day reality for both physicians and patients, the face of medicine fundamentally changed.

In the context of such dramatic results, curing and fixing moved to front and center stage. The art and philosophy of palliative care began to fade as more aggressive, more "satisfying" modalities became more easily accessible. Instead of building on the palliative care lessons and teachings of the past, American medicine began to focus entirely on the newly acquired scientific knowledge and the instruments and techniques that went with it. Universities, medical schools, and residency and fellowship programs devoted almost all their attention to mechanisms of disease, evidence-based medicine, and the development of newer and better procedures. Symptom control and the alleviation of pain and suffering took a back seat to curative and technological care. The economic incentives, prestige, department chairs and deanships, went to those proficient in scientific and technological medicine.

We lost the concept that modern medicine cannot reverse the ravages of all diseases, and that death is a natural course of life. Scientific and technological skills should in no way exclude skills in maximizing symptom and pain control. No matter what the disease process is, every patient should have the maximum available symptom and pain control. Every patient should be made as comfortable as possible, and consultation with physicians having excellent palliative care skills should be available to all.[1]

Dr. Cicely Saunders, who formalized the concept of hospice in 1967, was one of the few voices that confronted the need for compassionate, palliative care during the scientific and medical technology boom. However, programs like hospice as we know it today did not come to the forefront until the 1980s. The medical profession is starting to face the need for hospice now, but we still have a long way to go.

DEATH SCARES PEOPLE. SO DOES GRIEF

Grief avoidance can be a problem when a family member is in an end-of-life situation. Often, families insist on intrusive, painful, even disfiguring care for a patient at the end of life who would only benefit from palliative and hospice care. The death of a loved one is permanent and painful, and many of us simply don't even want to think about grieving. "Grief Is A Journey Too" was a headline of a recent large city newspaper article.[2] The article contained family testimonials, reading lists, and other information to help its readers deal with grief. The fact that a major city newspaper would sense the need to publish an article like this is pretty strong proof that many of us have a problem with grieving.

Advance directives were mentioned in the article as a way to make the whole dying process less painful for both the patient and the family. As we have seen, however, they've turned out to be fool's gold in many cases. Most people don't even have them, and in the cases where they do, they often can't be found at the crucial time. It's somewhat foolish to ask people to make decisions about their care years in advance. Advance directives make no distinction between what is appropriate care for a 40-year-old who was in excellent health before an automobile accident and now requires intensive care and a respirator for a limited period of time from what is appropriate for a 90-year-old with metastatic cancer and renal failure who has no chance of survival at all. These kinds of decisions require an understanding of technical terms that are foreign to

Sometimes families insist on nonbeneficial care for a dying loved one to put off the grieving process as long as possible.

most people. All the complex and confusing language may inadvertently nurture the fantasy that death is an option that can be avoided.

As discussed in Chapter 2, treatment choices should be confined to those options that are appropriate to the patient's overall condition. However, it seems that a lot of technological and procedural end-of-life care is driven by the desire to postpone death and grieving to the last possible moment, even though it may cause the patient more pain and more discomfort, sometimes to the point of bodily desecration. It is troubling to watch a loving family misinterpret the Patient Self-Determination Act or the Americans with Disabilities Act, believing that they are protecting their family member by insisting on nonbeneficial care.

We often hear, "We want everything done," but what does that really mean? Is the general consensus that every conceivable technique should be undertaken regardless of the chances of success or the suffering it will cause the patient? Taken to the extreme, should organ transplants be performed in patients with widely metastatic cancer even though there is absolutely no chance of success? Or does "everything done" mean the best possible care after careful consideration of the overall condition of the patient?

There is a lot of confusion around this issue. Rational decisions about appropriate care get lost in the shuffle sometimes because:

- Physicians and hospitals benefit financially from providing more therapy, no matter how absurd.
- Many people have difficulty accepting the inevitability of death.
- There is always the specter of legal action hovering in the background.

The *Gilgunn v. Massachusetts General Hospital* case is classic example.[3]

When Does Doing Everything Possible for a Patient Become Inappropriate Care?

Mrs. Gilgunn was in an obvious end-of-life situation, but her daughter was under the impression that she wanted "everything done." The physicians and the ethics committee of the Mass General Hospital thought that meant, in this situation, the best possible palliative care and that Mrs. Gilgunn would not want to refuse that care. Her daughter interpreted her mother's request as meaning that the respirator and artificial feeding should be continued indefinitely. The physicians instituted end-of-life palliative care, and shortly thereafter Mrs. Gilgunn died. The daughter sued, and the trial judge found in favor of the physicians and the hospital.

There were those, of course, who felt the physicians had abandoned the patient and had shown no respect for Mrs. Gilgunn as a human being, Actually, it was just the opposite. The staff of Massachusetts General Hospital was advocating for the patient, and the only way for Mrs. Gilgunn to retain any sense of humanity was to recognize that she was in an end-of-life situation, and that the best possible palliative care would be respecting her wishes that "everything be done." The options for the daughter were either to accept her wishes to receive the best palliative care, or to ignore her mother's request, refuse that care, and let her die without comfort care. Either way, there was no turning back for Mrs. Gilgunn.

PAIN CONTROL AND COMFORT CARE AT THE END OF LIFE

The concept of physician-assisted suicide is a reflection of the failure of physicians to provide satisfactory end-of-life care. Patients should not suffer, and families should not have to deplete their live savings on inappropriate care. Pain at the end of life can be treated, and in 90 percent of the cases well controlled.[4] Symptom control is paramount and includes control of pain, depression, and anxiety. Recognizing that an end-of-life situation is at hand and replacing curative care with excellent palliative care and hospice can save vast amounts of resources, both financial and emotional.

The American Pain Society has published a recent article to help physicians provide excellent pain control.[5] Palliative sedation is available for the 10 percent of patients at the end of their lives for whom even the best pain management does not control symptoms or bring comfort.[6] The U.S. Supreme Court has ruled that if the intent of treatment is the relief of suffering and not to induce death, terminal sedation is an acceptable form of treatment.[7]

Modern medicine has many excellent tools to control pain at the end of life.

Patients in severe pain live somewhat longer with excellent pain control. These patients are definitely not candidates for cardiopulmonary resuscitation. As with any other rational therapy, the patient/family has the right to refuse optimal pain therapy, but this would be extremely rare.

THE BIRTH OF HOSPICE IN AMERICA

hos·pice (hsps): Noun, from Old French adaptation of Latin *hospitium*, meaning hospitality. 1. Originally referred to places that took in travelers, or places of shelter for the poor maintained by various monastic orders. 2. Today, it refers to programs that provide palliative care for end-of-life patients in their homes, inpatient facilities, or free-standing hospice facilities.

As I mentioned at the beginning of this chapter, before World War II and the scientific advances that followed, doctors did palliative care and hospice-type work with their patients in their homes. These compassionate skills began to fade as doctors had to focus more and more on the new knowledge that was transforming medicine.

Visitors from overseas first brought the concept of hospice to the United States. Dr. Cecily Saunders was a nurse in England who went on to become a physician, and founded hospice in 1967. When she was invited to speak at the Yale School of Nursing in 1965, she brought the experience of hospice care to a whole new generation of nurses.

Another pioneer in end-of-life care was Dr. Elisabeth Kübler-Ross, a Swiss physician who emigrated to the United States in 1958. She was appalled by the treatment of dying patients in hospitals,[8] and wrote the book *On Death and Dying* in 1969. She testified before the U.S. Senate Special Committee on Aging in 1972.

It wasn't long before the ball really got rolling with hospice care:

1974: The National Cancer Institute funded the New Haven Hospice. New Haven Hospice created the ten principles of hospice care.[9]

1. Patients and family is the unit of care.
2. Physicians direct and nurses coordinate care.
3. Symptom control is paramount—physical, psychological, spiritual, and sociological.
4. Care is via an interdisciplinary team
5. With volunteers.
6. On a 365-days-a-year basis.
7. Follow-up for bereavement is available for the family.
8. Home and in-patient care are a continuum.
9. Ability to pay is not a barrier.
10. Emotional support for the staff is ongoing.

1978: The U.S. National Hospice Organization was established. The U.S. Department of Health, Education and Welfare certified that hospice care is a viable alternative for individuals with terminal illnesses. With that endorsement, the National Cancer Institute funded more hospices in California, Arizona, and New Jersey between 1978 and 1980.

1980: A 44-bed inpatient hospice unit was created in the Yale-New Haven hospital.

1982: Congress passed a Medicare Hospice Benefit. The Arthur Vining Foundation provided funding to promote spirituality within the hospice movement.

1988: Physicians founded the American Academy of Hospice and Palliative Medicine as a movement for physicians to return to their roots and reemphasize that physicians' primary responsibility is to relieve pain and suffering. Sometimes that means curing disease, sometimes it means controlling disease, and sometimes it means just letting go and focusing entirely on symptoms and pain control. The goal is always to minimize pain and suffering.

1993: Certification for Hospice and Palliative Care Nursing was initiated.

2000: The National Hospice Organization changed its name to National Hospice and Palliative Care Organization and awarded the first winner of the Distinguished Award for Outstanding Research in Hospice and Palliative Care. The Robert Wood Johnson Foundation funded national comprehensive education to improve end-of-life care by nurses, based on the pioneering work at the New Haven Hospice.

HOSPICE TODAY

Hospice is a concept of care, not necessarily a specific place of care, although the number of free-standing hospice facilities is growing. The focus of hospice is palliative rather than curative treatment and on quality of life rather than length of life. Sophisticated symptom relief is provided through professional medical care, and both patient and family are included in the care. Trained volunteers can offer respite care for family members as well as meaningful support to the patient.

Hospice looks at dying as a normal process of life, and the care neither hastens nor postpones death. Each dying person has a variety of physical, spiritual, emotional, and social needs. So does the family. Each is so unique that the goal of the hospice team is to be sensitive and responsive to the special requirements of each individual patient and family.

Hospice care is provided to patients who have a limited life expectancy. Most hospice patients are cancer patients, but hospice accepts anyone regardless of age or illness. All of these patients have made the decision to spend their last months at home or in a homelike setting. Hospice patients receive care in their personal residences, nursing homes, hospital hospice units, and in-patient hospice centers. Hospice workers assess the patient and family situation, make arrangements for any special equipment that might be needed, and counsel family and friends about care giving.

The "Who" of Hospice

Hospice care is based on teamwork. The team usually includes a physician, a nurse, a home health aide, a social worker, a chaplain, and a volunteer. Consultations with the patient and the family about their unique needs dictate the make-up of the team.

Only one-fifth of end-of-life patients receive hospice care. The other four-fifths die in institutions, frequently with no comfort or palliative care, often isolated and alone.

Under the direction of the patient's physician, a hospice nurse makes regularly scheduled visits to the patient to provide pain management and symptom control. The nurse keeps the primary physician informed of the patient's condition. Nurses provide a full compliment of skilled nursing care and are available 24 hours a day, seven days a week.

Home health aides provide assistance with the personal care of the patient. This might include bathing, changing the sheets, feeding, or sometimes just reading to them.

Social workers deal with more practical, logistical, and financial issues, as well as lending emotional support, providing counseling and bereavement follow-up. They assess the need for volunteers and other support services needed by the family, and help get the family and community support services together.

Chaplains provide spiritual support to patients and families and serve as a bridge between them and their religious community. Chaplains often assist with memorial services and funeral arrangements.

An Enlightened Family

A 90-year-old gentleman, fortunate to have the support of a loving family so he could live at home, had a history of coronary heart disease, moderate dementia, and deafness. Because of severe abdominal pain, he was admitted to a community hospital. He was found to be hypotensive (low blood pressure) with a rigid abdomen, deteriorating kidney function, severe acidosis (liver and kidneys unable to deal with the acids generated by his tissues), and suspected bacteria in his blood stream (sepsis). He was given antibiotics, and a diagnosis of ischemic (not enough blood supply) bowel disease was made. Over the ensuing two days, his renal function continued to deteriorate, and acidosis became more severe. His daughter was on dialysis, so the family was familiar with the rigors of this procedure. Because of his age, worsening kidney function and frail state of health, the surgeons felt that he could not survive an operation to remove the segment of ischemic bowel. He would also need acute dialysis, but the ischemic bowel problem would still be an issue. Both he and his family agreed that the appropriate course of action was palliative care and hospice. The medical team agreed and supported their choice. After three days in the hospital, he was discharged to an independent hospice facility where he died (with no CPR) four days later, surrounded by family, in no pain, and as comfortable as possible.

Comfort and Pain Management

Patients choose hospice because they want to be with family and friends but still be comfortable and as pain-free as possible. Hospice can help them reach this goal with the latest medications and devices for pain relief that still allow the patient to be alert and interacting with family. Physical and occupational therapists help many patients to be as mobile and self-sufficient as they wish. In many cases, depending on location, specialists in music therapy, art therapy, massage, and diet counseling are also available. Knowing that emotional and spiritual health can make a big difference in the quality of the patient's life, various counselors, including clergy, are available to assist family members as well as patients.

Who Pays for the Hospice Services?

Hospice is covered by Medicare nationwide, by Medicaid in 41 states, and by most private insurance companies. Medicare covers all services and supplies for the hospice patient related to the terminal illness. Medicare reimbursement rules ask for two physicians to declare that the patient has six months or less to live, although payment continues if the estimate is incorrect and the patient lives longer. The physician declaration is taken to mean that the patient would not benefit from readmission to an acute care hospital to attempt cure, but could be admitted for symptom relief. In some hospices, the patient may be required to pay a 5 percent or $5 co-payment on medication and a 5 percent co-payment for respite care. If someone has no coverage of any kind and cannot pay, most hospices will provide services using money raised from the community or from memorial or foundation gifts.

DOES USING HOSPICE SAVE MONEY?

There is some debate about whether hospice care is less costly, although there is no doubt than it is more appropriate and humane. One study found that hospice costs less for patients on a quick trajectory to death with a cancer diagnosis, more for patients with an intermediate course with organ failure, and the highest cost for patients with a long course such as with dementia.[10] This study was retrospective using administrative Medicare data and not chart reviews, and may reflect the longer life span when hospice is used instead of being reflective of attempts at curative care and the unintended consequence of increased mortality. This question cannot be definitively answered until there is a prospective case-controlled study comparing patients assigned to hospice, preferably at home, to those in the same state of health dying in institutions, especially acute care hospitals. It is doubtful if a study of this nature will ever be undertaken.

Financial comparisons are difficult to make because the retrospective Medicare administrative data does not take into account the reasons why some patients chose hospice and others did not. However, if end-of-life patients were not in Intensive Care Units, were not recycled from nursing home to hospital and back, and did not receive operations and chemotherapy before death, there is no doubt that not only would end-of-life care be of higher quality but costs would be significantly lower.

The percentage of total Medicare expenditures during the last year of life has remained constant at about 27 percent. Fifty-two percent of this amount is spent during the last 60 days of life.[11] More recently, studies show expenses during the last year of life were 22 percent of all medical expenditures, 26 percent of Medicare costs, 18 percent of all non-Medicare costs, and 25 percent of Medicaid costs.[12]

Since hospice use has also increased during this same period, one could argue that hospice has not led to significantly lower end-of-life costs. However with the increased use of ICUs and technology for most patients at the end of life, the more likely argument is that the increase in technological deaths, with their high associated costs, have offset the savings created by hospice use.

Others have argued that controlling end-of-life costs is a conflict between economics and bioethics. Economics, they say, is concerned about the production, distribution and consumption of goods, while bioethics focuses on competing values without regard to cost.[13] However, with Appropriate Care Committees helping physicians make good decisions, there would be no conflict. Treating patients inappropriately at the end of life with acute care and technology is not only unethical, it is wasteful. Every patient who has any chance of improvement should be treated with all available tools, but patients who have no chance of benefit should not be subjected to inappropriate, expensive technology.

We are witnessing one of the great American tragedies. One-fifth of patients in end-of-life care situations are in a hospice setting and receiving excellent palliative care. Four-fifths die in an institution with poor palliation, and in many cases, are alone. Frequently families believe they are defending their loved one by insisting they receive technological/curative acute care. However, when patients cannot benefit because of their overall general condition, they can only be harmed by inappropriate care. The voices calling for appropriate, compassionate end-of-life care have been growing for many years. In 1997, Howard Brody and colleagues wrote: "Forced to choose between what they were trained to do and what they were never trained to do, physicians and nurses may continue aggressive therapy well beyond the point at which patients or families (or the healthcare professionals themselves) would prefer to stop."[14]

Follow-up of 2,607 patients with either chronic obstructive pulmonary disease (COPD), congestive heart failure (CHF), or end-stage liver disease demonstrated that recommended clinical criteria were unable to predict with accuracy when a patient would die.[15] But the physicians *were* able to determine that palliative care and hospice, and not acute hospital procedural and technological care, were the treatments of choice. This further illustrates that it is quite difficult to predict how long a patient will live. However, the critical determination in light of the overall condition of the patient is that attempts at curative care in an acute care hospital are not beneficial, and the patient is best served by end-of-life palliative care and hospice.

CHAPTER 8

A Big Step in the Right Direction: The VA Transforms End-of-Life Care

Some people will think the ideas presented in this book so far are impractical or even pie in the sky. What follows is proof that the healthcare system can provide humane, end-of-life care. It is material from a short Veterans Administration Handbook called *The VA Transforms End-of-Life Care.**

I extend my deepest thanks to all the people involved in putting together the handbook and for allowing me to use the material in this chapter. At the end of this chapter is a listing of all the people involved in creating the handbook and contacts for getting a copy. I would like to add an additional thank you to Diane Jones of Ethos Consulting, and Dr. Scott Shreve, National Director of Hospice and Palliative Care Services for the VA.

After reading the handbook, I was impressed at the care and thought that had gone into developing the VA's end-of-life program over the years, and how they are continually monitoring, revising, and improving it to provide the most compassionate care while wisely using resources.

It is an ever-evolving program, and there are many lessons to be learned by their example. The VA is an enormous organization, yet they have done a masterful job of coordinating resources, both human and financial, within the VA and local communities to make sure that veterans receive appropriate, caring support at the end of their lives.

The VA has demonstrated what can successfully be done on a large scale. Perhaps this presents an excellent challenge to healthcare institutions all over the United States to reassess their own programs (or lack of same), and rise to the challenge of providing the very best care for end-of-life patients, and the best use of resources all around.

---

*Beresford, Larry, The VA Transforms End-of-Life Care, compiled for the Veterans Administration, 2005. In the public domain.

THE VA TRANSFORMS END-OF-LIFE CARE FOR VETERANS

Stephen Pavon served in the Marine Corps Air Wing from 1963 to 1967, including a tour in Vietnam. While on active convoy duty, he was injured twice, patched up and sent back out. During the "times of turmoil" that followed his discharge, Pavon was a fireman, a college student, and a hippie in Berkeley, Calif. Later, he taught transcendental meditation, traveled the world, and worked overseas as an engineer before finally landing as a horse trainer on a ranch in Nevada. Now Pavon, 57, is fighting another battle, one he will not win, against rectal cancer. He will spend his final days at the Veterans Affairs Palo Alto Health Care System in Palo Alto, Calif., where Dr. James Hallenbeck, Director of Palo Alto's Palliative Care Services, and his team are building and refining a new model of expert, compassionate, supportive care for veterans nearing the end of their lives. "I've never heard a 'no' here," Pavon reports. "The support is so complete that it allows me to be comfortable and to live my final days in comfort. I get to personalize my room. I can still maintain control of my heart, my mind, and my intelligence."

When the 25-bed Palo Alto Hospice Care Center was created in 1979, it was at the vanguard of a national hospice movement that would transform care for dying people nationwide. Today, the Hospice Care Center remains at the forefront of innovation. It received a 2001 Citation of Honor through the American Hospital Association's Circle of Life Awards for exemplary end-of-life care. It is also the hub site for a network of six interdisciplinary hospice and palliative care fellowship training programs within the VA.

The unit's staff includes psychologists, a half-time massage therapist, and 25 volunteers, in addition to the requisite hospice doctors, nurses, social worker, and chaplain. Families, who often travel to be near a loved one, may stay overnight on rollout beds or in free facilities on the hospital's campus, says Hallenbeck, who, in addition to his role at the hospice care center is assistant professor of medicine at nearby Stanford University.

VA PROGRAMS TREAT BODY, MIND, AND SPIRIT

Hospice care, whether it is provided inpatient in VA medical centers or in patients' private residences by partnering community hospice programs, combines expert symptom management and pain relief with compassionate attention to the psychological and spiritual dimensions and family dynamics that arise when confronting a terminal illness. Quality of life becomes paramount when its quantity is limited. Hospice also supports grieving family members for a year or more after the patient's death.

For the national VA health system, recent advances in developing, refining and expanding hospice and palliative care, an approach aimed at bringing hospice's holistic, comfort-oriented care philosophy to seriously ill patients earlier in their disease progression, are not mere frills. That is because an estimated 1,600 veterans die every day in this country, most of them members of the Greatest Generation who won World War II. Now in their 80s, they are nearing the end of their natural life spans. Veterans account for 28 percent of all deaths in the United States in 2004.

Through a national network of state and local Hospice-Veteran Partnerships, VA is sharing what it has learned about such care with the community agencies that provide the majority of hospice care to terminally ill veterans.

Hospice-Veteran Partnerships are part of a system-wide transformation aimed at honoring veterans' preferences for care at the end of life, says Dr. Thomas Edes, who is VA's chief administrator overseeing this transformation. In response to increasing and changing demands for end-of-life services, VA has issued a number of recent directives mandating hospice and palliative care.

"We now have a framework and a structure in place," Edes says. "All of the pieces are aligned. Hospice is now a covered benefit for all enrolled veterans, home hospice care is in the VA budget for the first time, and we have a national standard for purchasing hospice care from community providers. We can track hospice workload for resource allocation and planning, and we have a hospice point of contact at every VA facility. We want to elevate expectations and make it easy for veterans to access hospice and palliative care."

While the largely autonomous local Veterans Administration Medical Centers (VAMCs) are given flexibility to address end-of-life care according to their veterans' needs, national policy and standards stipulate that each VA facility have the following resources and services:

- A designated hospice contact person who is part of an integrated network for local and national communications and information dissemination.
- Provision of needed hospice services in all settings.
- Inpatient hospice beds or access to them in the community.
- An interdisciplinary palliative care consultation team.
- Assistance with referrals to community hospices in its service area.
- Tracking of hospice and palliative care services provided to veterans in all settings.

In many cases, the local approach may include a dedicated hospice unit, such as at the Palo Alto VAMC, based in either a hospital or an extended care facility. Palliative care teams may consult on pain and symptom management for outpatient clinics as well as throughout the hospital. VA's own home-based primary care or specialized geriatric services may also be involved in developing end-of-life care programs.

"We will institutionalize, in the best sense of the word, hospice and palliative care in the largest integrated health system in the world, proactively creating an end-of-life care system while implementing permanent changes, making it an integral part of the fabric of what VA is," says palliative care consultant Diane Jones. That kind of integration has not yet happened in the private sector, she notes, even though U.S. hospices will care for 900,000 dying patients in 2004.

"We're doing a lot of things to bolster that institutionalization . . . a lot of program development, a lot of action. The challenge now is to create an enduring network of skilled, trained, committed professionals," Edes adds. "It's our privilege and our responsibility to ensure that veterans receive comfort, support and care as they face their final days and that they have a choice of where they receive this care. Some don't. I am concerned that in the past far too many veterans have suffered quietly, graciously accepting far less than the services they rightly deserve."

Although much has been accomplished in the last few years, more must be done to consolidate and sustain the gains at every level. The VA's newly established ability to measure and track the types of end-of-life care being provided in each facility—the workload—is a major step forward. Changing the medical culture from top to bottom at each facility is another significant challenge. VA leaders aim to create an environment in which VAMC staff are comfortable referring patients to hospice and palliative care and bringing up death and dying as part of routine advance care planning conversations with seriously ill veterans and their families.

"Is there a well-functioning palliative care team at every facility, as we have mandated? Are those teams adequately trained and staffed? At this point, probably not," Edes concedes. "But we are raising expectations at the national and local levels, so that a terminally ill veteran can go to any VA facility and obtain hospice care. If needed hospice care is not forthcoming, we want them to contact us. And we now have champions working in every VA facility, so we are getting closer to our target."

Stephen Pavon says he has encountered the VA health system twice in his life, and both experiences were positive. The first time, five years ago, he was referred to a post-traumatic stress disorder (PTSD) program at the nearby Menlo Park VA outpatient clinic.

"That saved my life. The communication skills they gave me helped me clean up my life," he says. After five failed marriages and multiple job changes, "I had turned isolation into a profession."

More recently, Pavon was living on his isolated Nevada ranch where a hospice team from Barton Memorial Hospital in South Lake Tahoe, Calif., visited and cared for him. When he could no longer manage living alone, even with the help of friends, "they had a room waiting for me here on the VA hospice unit." Before entering, Pavon wrapped up his personal business, found a good home for his horse, gave away his golf clubs and conga drums, and paid all of his bills—including a prepaid cremation service.

When he came to the Palo Alto VA hospice unit, he expected to find the same level of compassionate, spiritually oriented, medically expert hospice care that he had received from Barton Hospice—and he has. Sitting in his hospice room, wearing his black cowboy hat, Pavon reflects on a restless but full life and on the cancer that has come to dominate but not define his final days.

Mellow and sanguine about his prospects, Pavon could be a spokesperson for the hospice philosophy. "The whole underlying theme here is my comfort. I'm under 24-hour care and they've got me covered. If something isn't working, they come in and fix it and I'm back on the road. Medically, they're all up to snuff. They know how to give me the tools I need and they don't stop until I'm in my comfort zone," he says.

Pavon observes, "Sometimes, you find a simple word that explains you. I can relate my whole current existence, my spirituality, anything, to that concept of comfort." People are born into this world in need of comfort, he says. Sometimes, at the end, they need more help to maintain a degree of comfort, and that's where hospice comes in.

In Pavon's case, a percutaneous infusion catheter (PIC) and portable pump deliver high doses of Dilaudid, a powerful synthetic form of morphine that keeps his pain under control without sacrificing his lucidness.

"I've had great adventures. Sometimes I wish I'd stayed a fireman—a nice, steady job," Pavon says. "But I traveled all over the world. I was always trying to fit in— trying to find where I belonged."

* * *

Another celebrated VA hospice unit opened almost a decade ago at the Bay Pines VAMC in St. Petersburg, Fla. Clinical coordinator Deborah Grassman, a nurse practitioner, is an impassioned advocate for understanding and meeting the unique needs of combat veterans and their families. The 10-bed unit dispenses human kindness to facilitate opportunities for terminally ill veterans on the unit to die healed, in comfort and at peace. For example, the hospice unit does not restrict visiting hours—or even types of visitors, who often include young children or family pets. The unit gives families a toll-free number they can call for medical updates.

Visiting children may play in a children's room whenever a break is needed for the patient or child. Disabled vets may explore the hospital grounds using motorized wheelchairs. A whirlpool bubble bath with hydraulic lift and the staff's use of healing touch modalities also enhance patients' quality of life. Hospice gives each family a "Comfort Cart" laden with aromatherapy supplies, massage oils, recorded music, and other aids for making the environment seem less institutional.

The hospice team holds weekly "quality-of-life" meetings with patients, family members and staff to discuss how to keep patients and families comfortable, using that input to shape the care provided by the hospice team. The character of the unit is also reflected in a cooked-to-order breakfast served each Wednesday to patients and families on the unit by Chaplain Dan Hummer and hospice volunteers.

Special "eleventh hour" volunteers can be called in to keep vigil for dying patients who would otherwise spend their final hours alone. One of these volunteers, Judy Dellerba, says, "I feel it is an honor and privilege to be there with them." Dellerba's own husband died on the unit two years ago, and the hospice grief support program helped her through the period following his death.

MEETINGS WITHOUT AGENDAS

John Cornhoff, an 87-year-old World War II veteran dying of end-stage dementia and pneumonia, is surrounded by several generations of his family, from children to a great-grandchild. Those not present in person have been brought in by speakerphone. Hospice staff members join them for a quality-of-life meeting.

"We gather like this to be with you and hear what's on your hearts and minds. We don't have an agenda," Grassman begins. Cornhoff's boisterous, obviously loving family recently made the decision not to have a tube inserted through his nose into his stomach for artificial nutrition and hydration. Grassman suggests that their decision may be helping him to die more peacefully. She points out that he now seems to be turning inward, a sign of approaching death.

"The body has its own wisdom," she says. "We're just honoring what's happening to John, a very holy process to which we want to bring dignity."

Each of Cornhoff's assembled loved ones speaks in turn to reminisce and say goodbye with a mixture of laughter and tears. "Dad has always lived life to the fullest," says older daughter Peggy, who sits on her father's bed to be near him. "He taught us to enjoy life and each other. He accepts people the way they are. We go forward, we don't go backward."

Over the speakerphone, son-in-law Tom asks, "Are you listening to this, Dad?" Eyes closed, mouth open, laboring over each breath, head bent on the pillow, Cornhoff nods perceptibly. Someone describes this to Tom, who jokes, "Can I have the ten bucks you owe me?"

In another room on the unit, another patient's family has a smaller, more subdued quality-of-life meeting. Matthew Civilette, 77, and his only living daughter, Fran, meet with the hospice team. Civilette, who has kidney cancer, saw extensive action in the Philippines during World War II. With a resigned look on his face, Civilette says he's ready, almost impatient to die. Just a week ago, he was up, and dancing at the assisted living facility where he had been living.

"The quicker I go, the better. I've had a good life. I'm 77 years old. Nobody escapes," he says. "We had breakfast together this morning at quarter to six, my usual time," Civilette informs the team, nodding to his daughter.

"They promised scrambled eggs and toast and they delivered." "And he sat up and ate them," Fran adds. After a bit of reflection, she says, "I'm upset about losing my dad, but it happens to all of us. What can you do?"

"I'll still talk to you after, if I can figure out how," Civilette tells his daughter. "I'm glad you brought me here [to the hospice unit]. It's very pleasant." The next day, Civilette died in the way he had hoped: peacefully, quickly, and with his daughter at his side. Grassman later reported, "Fran touched him and told him that she loved him as he took his last breath."

SHARED VISION, SHARED WORK: VA AND ITS HOSPICE PARTNERS

Under the leadership of CEO Mary Labyak, The Hospice of the Florida Suncoast (The Hospice) has become the largest and best-known nonprofit hospice program in the country, serving some 1,600 terminally ill patients each day. From its Pinellas County headquarters, The Hospice operates a national education institute and provides a broad range of community outreach programs, successfully weaving its care into the fabric of the retirement communities of greater St. Petersburg. The communities it serves also lie within the service area of Bay Pines VAMC. Although both groups share similar goals, until recently, they had not mapped out ways to work together and learn from one another.

The realization that this was necessary came when Deborah Grassman gave her groundbreaking educational presentation on the different experiences and needs of combat veterans at the end of life to staff at The Hospice. Many staff had not realized that veterans had unique experiences and needs, and that care could be designed to accommodate those needs.

"You see people with 20 to 25 years of hospice experience—like me—realizing that there are big parts of people's lives we somehow missed," Labyak says. "There needs to be a call to action for hospices about why the unique needs of veterans are important," Labyak says. "It's not just about reimbursement. It's a huge step forward for access and quality for community hospices just to be having the conversation with VA about what's different for veterans.

"Precipitated by Deborah's phenomenal presentation, we have started thinking here in new ways about patients in pain, about terminal restlessness. It has become a wonderful learning experience for us, tapping a rich new vein for our professional practice and reinforcing our mission."

The Hospice of the Florida Suncoast and the Bay Pines VA hospice unit have developed their relationship, working through designated staff liaisons and learning from each other, says program director Marcie Pruitt. Primary care physicians at Bay Pines can refer to The Hospice, and its after-hours physician coverage, without having to sever their link to their patients, while Bay Pines contracts with The Hospice to offer bereavement support group on the unit. A key focus for their collaboration is managing the transition of veterans who are referred to The Hospice for care at home but eventually return to Bay Pines VAMC for longer-term inpatient care on its hospice unit.

An example of such give-and-take is Paxson (Pax) Parsons, a 55-year-old Vietnam veteran who is dying of lung cancer. Parsons is enrolled with The Hospice and receiving care at a quintessential Florida ranch-style house that he bought and refurbished shortly before his cancer was diagnosed. He lives alone, visited by a circle of friends, but plans to return to the Bay Pines hospice unit when he gets closer to the end. Parsons explains his plans and his history with the VA on a visit to his home with his hospice counselor, Harriet Hoke.

He projects a striking image with his shaved head, piercing eyes, rainbow striped kimono, gold neck chains and a nasal cannula hooked around his ears. The cannula is attached to an enormous length of rubber tubing, which allows him to wander freely around his house and back to his pool while remaining connected to the oxygen dispenser.

A PAINFUL EYE OPENER

Parsons was 21 years old when he was sent to Vietnam. "When we were flying in, they told us to put our heads down. Well, it is a big deal when you start getting shot at," he says. Parsons returned stateside in 1970 with physical and psycho-logical disabilities that required care from VA. In those days, he says, "You really had to fight for what you needed."

Indeed, Parson was eventually confined to a psychiatric hospital and later treated for drug addiction. He has been in recovery for 20 years and is enrolled in a VA stress management program for PTSD. "I've gotten better thanks to the Bay Pines VAMC. They helped me because they treated me like a person," he observes.

"My life really began after Vietnam. 'Nam was bad, but it opened my eyes," Parsons says. "Once you've been in a war zone, your life changes like that [snap]. I was born Southern Baptist and I was gay. Surprisingly, my family is very accept-ing of me now. I love who I am and who I became. Even my two daughters have come a long way with that," he relates.

"I went into the Carolina Mountains, got my life together and got off drugs," he continues. He explored spiritual traditions, including Native American heal-ing—he's part Cherokee—spirit guides and the 12-step acknowledgement of a higher power. "I discovered a whole new me—Pax, not Paxson. I left Paxson back in Vietnam. He's scary. You don't want to meet him," he warns.

Eventually, Parsons took charge of his own life, helping to establish an HIV volunteer program in Delaware in the 1980s. This experience of working with dying people changed his view of dying. "That's why I'm not afraid of death. Be-cause of the whole war issue and what I went through, it made me feel the pain of other people," he says.

Parsons has since helped many veterans negotiate their benefits and complete the necessary paperwork to obtain VA services, while supporting others to be-come more accepting of who they are.

He encourages other veterans with life-threatening illnesses to be open to hospice care. "It's a lifeline," he says. You'll be a lot more comfortable. It's not about dying—that part's up to you. Hospice is just a helping hand, helping you live with the disease. It's helped me a lot."

Epilogue: Pax Parsons never made it to the Bay Pines VAMC unit. His lung cancer advanced more quickly than expected, so his partner, Don, and his sister, who was staying with him, decided to try to keep him at home. On March 14, a month after the writer's visit, he was still up and walking around the serene, art-filled home that gave him so much comfort, although increased breathing diffi-culties and inability to swallow pills signaled a decline. The next day he died at home, comfortably and relatively free of pain, in the company of loved ones and attended by his spirit guides.

Across the country on May 26, Stephen Pavon died on the hospice unit at the Palo Alto VAMC, peacefully and comfortably.

Now that you've read the story of the VA's end-of-life care program, the big question is, how did they do it? The most impressive part of the plan-ning is that they reached out to and enlisted the assistance of many diverse groups and individuals. Each brought ideas and perspectives and in some cases funding, helped build the foundation of the program, ensure its sustainability, and provide for its growth and expansion. One of the most powerful aspects of their efforts is the coordination of community services in outlying localities with services and needs within the VA program. As you read through these next sections, note the diversity of the players and the actions taken, and the care and thought that was put into creating programs that meet the needs of dying veterans. There is a wealth of information that could provide the beginnings of a blueprint for end-of-life care reform in the private sector as well.

VA AT THE VANGUARD OF IMPROVING END-OF-LIFE CARE

Individual champions and facilities have advocated for hospice care in VA since the earliest days of the American hospice movement in the 1970's. National efforts to expand those isolated incidents into a more systematic approach to end-of-life care for the VA system received an important boost from Dr. Kenneth Kizer, VA Under Secretary for Health from 1994 to 1999. Different departments within VA's central office, including the Office of Academic Affiliations (OAA); Geriatrics and Extended Care Strategic Healthcare Group and Home and Community-Based Care, both within the Office of Patient Care Services; and Employee Education System, have made significant contributions to the emergence of a more comprehensive and coordinated approach to end-of-life care within VA.

In 1997, Kizer convened a VA End-of-Life Summit, bringing together experts and advocates to explore the issues. This led to the development of national outcomes measures reflecting greater accountability for appropriate end-of-life care; among these was the "Pain as a Fifth Vital Sign" initiative, an effort in which VA led the nation in recognizing and treating pain.

Since then, VA has conducted several projects aimed at improving quality, enhancing training and education for physicians and others involved in end-of-life care, and coordinating VA hospice and palliative care services. Funded in part from generous grants from national organizations interested in improving end-of-life care, they are:

- **VA Faculty Leader Project for Improved Care at the End of Life,** funded in part by a generous grant from the Robert Wood Johnson Foundation, identified and supported 30 faculty leaders to establish palliative care training curriculums within the VAMC-based internal medicine residency programs. As a reminder, VAMC stands for Veterans Administration Medical Center.
- **Training and Program Assessment for Palliative Care (TAPC),** supported by the Office of Academic Affiliations, included a national survey to identify and describe actual end-of life care practices in VAMCs.
- **Interprofessional Fellowship Program in Palliative Care.** Administered by the Office of Academic Affiliations, these clinically focused fellowships

are based at six competitively chosen VAMCs with experience in providing palliative care and each include one or two VA in the Vanguard of Improving End-of-Life-Care physicians and two or three other health professionals. The hub for the fellowship network, in Palo Alto, Calif., also supports a Web-based VA Nationwide Palliative Care Network.

- **VA Hospice and Palliative Care Initiative,** a two-year effort bringing together more than 40 VA and community leaders to design programs that would accelerate access to compassionate and coordinated hospice and palliative care services for all veterans. Rallying Points, a national program of Last Acts Partnership for Caring, joined with VA to extend VAHPC beyond its initial two years. Seed money was provided by the National Hospice and Palliative Care Organization and the Center for Advanced Illness Coordinated Care.
- **National Hospice-Veteran Partnership Program** supported in part by Rallying Points, is actively promoting national, state and local collaborations among VAMCs, community hospices and other partnering groups to improve access to hospice and palliative care for all veterans.
- **Accelerated Administrative and Clinical Training (AACT),** supported by Geriatrics and Extended Care in collaboration with the Employee Education System and the Office of Academic Affiliations, is a program designed to disseminate the knowledge being gathered through VA's end-of-life initiatives. AACT brought together and trained multidisciplinary teams from each of the 21 VA VISNs (Veterans Integrated Service Networks) to encourage palliative care program development in their networks.

VA is now working to hire central office staff dedicated to hospice and palliative care development. The first of three projected central office staff, Dr. Scott Shreve, began as National Director of Hospice and Palliative Care Services in June 2004. Shreve is continuing to work half time as medical director of the hospice unit at the VAMC in Lebanon, Penn., while promoting quality improvement throughout VA. Resources: To view the Nationwide Palliative Care Network Web site and newsletter, go to www.hospice.va.gov. That site also contains a copy of the TAPC report. The TAPC toolkit and other end-of-life educational information are on the OAA Web site: www.va.gov/oaa/flp.

HOSPICE-VETERAN PARTNERSHIPS PROMOTE ACCESS

With support from VA headquarters, the National Hospice and Palliative Care Organization, the national Rallying Points office in Washington, D.C., the Center for Advanced Illness Coordinated Care in Albany, N.Y., and other end-of-life advocates, Hospice-Veteran Partnerships are now forming at state and regional levels to increase access to appropriate end-of-life care for veterans. They promote access by strengthening partnerships between VAMCs and their community partners, and by expanding their mutual knowledge base.

Some states are already well advanced in this dialogue while others are just starting to talk. A Hospice-Veteran Partnership "Toolkit" developed by the VA Hospice and Palliative Care Initiative and published by Rallying Points is full of suggestions for how to do this. Partnerships often are co-sponsored by state hospice organizations while bringing together community hospices, community end-of-life coalitions, veterans' service and alumni organizations, private service clubs, state Departments of Veterans Affairs, state veterans homes, the National Cemetery Association, local military treatment facilities, and VA professionals at the medical center and VISN levels.

"So much can be accomplished just by sitting around the table and talking with each other," says Kathleen Jacobs, Rallying Points Regional Resource Center Coordinator based at The Hospice of the Florida Suncoast in Largo. From there, coalitions typically assess unit local needs, develop a strategic plan for how best to serve veterans in the area, and then share information with veteran groups and the public. "Florida is a prototype of what can be done through partnerships," Jacobs says.

The Florida state group designed Hospice-Veteran Partnership commemorative pins with a card that reads, "Thank you . . . for your military service to America by advancing the universal hope of freedom and liberty for all." It distributed 20,000 of these pins in November 2003 to VA facilities, community hospices, veterans' organizations, and public officials, as well as at a number of commemorative events.

"These events helped to bring greater awareness to end-of-life issues and the need for advance care planning, without seeming morbid," says Joanne King, director of social work for Hospice of Volusia-Flagler in Port Orange and a member of the Hospice-Veteran Partnership of Florida. The coalition also co-sponsored a February 2004 statewide professional education teleconference on end-of-life care for veterans.

HOW CAN COMMUNITY HOSPICES COLLABORATE WITH VAMCs?

Approximately 3,200 hospice programs operate in the United States. Large and small, non-profit and for-profit, independent and hospital-based, they serve 900,000 terminally ill patients a year, most in private homes or in skilled nursing facilities. Hospices assist family caregivers, and eventually provide bereavement support to family survivors.

VA hospice units have learned a critical lesson in caring for dying veterans: a patient's military service history is highly relevant to providing the most appropriate, personalized end-of-life care. Although hospices routinely ask and record their patients' age, family make-up, racial/ethnic group and religion at the time of enrollment, few ask about service status. But they should. There may be health coverage and benefit issues, if the veteran is enrolled at a local VAMC or would like to be, along with burial and other benefits. In addition to exploring coverage status, hospices should consider incorporating the following questions into their admission process:

- Are you a veteran?
- Did you see combat?
- What was that like for you?
- Is there anything about your military experience that is still troubling to you?

The National Hospice and Palliative Care Organization (NHPCO) has long advocated that veterans should receive hospice care and that community hospices should be reimbursed by VA for the care they provide to appropriate, eligible veterans, says Judi Lund Person, NHPCO's Vice President for Quality End-of-Life Care. "NHPCO will continue to strongly support this work and relationship building as we look for funding opportunities to further advance the cause," she says.

In 2002 NHPCO contributed $100,000 to the VA Hospice and Palliative Care Initiative and today it plays an active leadership role in promoting Hospice-Veteran Partnerships nationwide. NHPCO recently awarded $5,000 grants to 10 state hospice and palliative care organizations to improve access to hospice care for veterans. Organizations in the Carolinas, Colorado, Connecticut, Illinois, Indiana, Kansas, Maine, Massachusetts, Michigan, and New York are integral parts of state Hospice Veteran Partnerships, working with VAMCs and other partners to assess the needs of dying veterans and provide hospice education and outreach.

"We have all of these dying veterans and we want to make their lives better. We want to figure out how to get community hospices more involved, and how to overcome barriers to coordinated care, so that we can provide the best end-of-life care for veterans and their families by whatever means necessary," Person says.

"It's not just about getting paid, but at the same time, that issue has been a sticking point for hospices. Now it's possible for VA to purchase hospice services from community hospices. But hospices need to understand that partnering is a two-way street," she explains. Hospices, which routinely market their services to health care facilities and providers, must do the same to encourage referrals from VAMCs.

"When I gave a keynote presentation to the California Hospice and Palliative Care Association last year, hospices wanted to know how to enter the 'impenetrable monolith' of VA—and how to find the right people within that system," says Dr. James Hallenbeck, Director of Palliative Care Services for the VA Palo Alto Health Care System. Although authorization for VA to pay for hospice care has existed for several years, individual programs may still encounter problems. These groups need to negotiate with VAMCs, using national guidelines, to work out kinks in the process at the local level.

Most important, Hallenbeck says, hospices should not approach VA as an insurance plan for covering hospice care in the community. They need to learn the subtleties of the relationship and recognize differences in language between the VA and Medicare.

"Hospices need to establish relationships and identify liaisons at both sides before individual coverage decisions are needed," he says. Find out which providers are dedicated to hospice and palliative care, and arrange to meet with them. The right person may be the palliative care consultation team coordinator, community health nurse or staff member on the hospice unit, if one exists in the facility.

"There are other nitty-gritty issues involved in the relationship, but these can be solved through conversation," Hallenbeck says. For example, VA physicians often are not accessible after 5 p.m. for emergency changes in medical orders. Since hospices require after-hours medical access, the hospice physician may assume this responsibility while preserving the VA primary care physician's involvement in the patient's care. These and other policy issues related to VAMCs working with community hospices are described in VA's new Handbook, "Procedures for Referral and Purchase of Community Hospice Care." The handbook is available on VA's publications Web page (www.va.gov/publ/direc/health/publications.asp).

WHAT'S DIFFERENT ABOUT DYING VETERANS?

Through her experience as clinical coordinator of the pioneering inpatient hospice unit at the Bay Pines VA Medical Center in St. Petersburg, Fla., Deborah Grassman has closely observed some important differences and lessons for providing end-of-life care to veterans. "It's only in the past ten years that we have started to realize that many things can influence a veteran's death," she says. Factors influencing veterans' experiences at the end of life include age, whether enlisted or drafted, branch of service, rank, and combat or POW experience.

Grassman presents a powerful and informative educational session on how health care professionals can attend to those differences. She has given the presentation to rapt professional audiences locally, nationally and in a recent VA educational teleconference.

"If veterans have seen combat, they have seen horrific things," Grassman says. Some are able to integrate that experience into their lives and as a result may be better equipped psychologically to cope with their own deaths. "These veterans are role models for how to have a good death, and in a death-denying society, that's important," she says. Still others suffer from post-traumatic stress disorder (PTSD), with symptoms that can include social isolation, alcohol abuse, and anxieties.

For some veterans, the effect of combat experience may remain buried for years, emerging only when the veteran is very sick and dying. In these cases, veterans may experience anxiety, agitation and resurrected memories connected to war experiences from many years before, Grassman says. Their medical caregivers need to differentiate these systems and treat them appropriately.

Doug Weadick, chaplain for the hospice unit at the Orlando, Fla., VA Health Center, has made similar observations. He notes, "When you're dying, you look back on significant events. Combat is a form of intimacy—very traumatic, life changing. It defined who they were and became. What I see is that they [veterans] want to process these events at the end of their lives."

Weadick says there is almost an audible sigh of relief for veterans who meet others like themselves on the hospice unit. "They're home—they're with people who have gone through the same things. They don't have to share their war stories. They just know the other person has gone down the same path."

Health professionals caring for veterans at the end of life should keep the following factors in mind:

- The demographics of veterans dying in the VA system, such as their higher degree of social isolation, lack of family support, or low income.
- The veteran's experience with military culture and the camaraderie of other veterans.
- A culture of stoicism that might prevent veterans from admitting to being in pain, or from asking for pain medication.
- The causes of terminal agitation, which may be related to PTSD or to disease-related terminal restlessness.
- Most dying people resist physical and chemical restraints—but for dying veterans, such restraints may be even more overwhelming.
- The possibility of paradoxical reactions to medications.

"I've seen many variations on these themes," says Dr. James Hallenbeck of the VA Palo Alto hospice unit. "I try to teach doctors on our unit to establish a relationship that starts with respect for the veteran. They were part of an experience that those who weren't there can't imagine. For a lot of our veterans, it's just polite to say, 'What branch of the service were you in?' If you acknowledge that aspect of their lives, you have a better chance of establishing respect and a connection," he says.

"Be careful of the stereotype of the homeless Vietnam veteran on the street— just like the stereotype that all World War II veterans are like John Wayne or Audie Murphy," Hallenbeck cautions. "Let's not overstate the case. Not every veteran suffered terrible trauma." What's needed now, he adds, is research to study further the anecdotal experiences coming out of VA hospice units and to connect that with VA system's extensive experience treating PTSD.

DEDICATION AND ACKNOWLEDGMENTS

We dedicate this monograph as a loving tribute to Marsha Goodwin, RN and MSN. The remarkable progress VA has made in advancing end-of-life care was made possible by the dedicated leadership and compassionate support of Marsha Goodwin. During her years in the Geriatric and Extended Care Strategic Healthcare Group in VA Central Office, Marsha provided skilled guidance, articulated core values and initiated enduring actions that led to the tremendous advances made throughout the nation to ensure access to hospice and palliative care for the veterans we are privileged to serve.

This report was developed by an editorial review committee consisting of Diane Jones, Thomas Edes, and Judi Lund Person. Editorial assistance was also provided by Don Mickey and Janice Lynch Schuster. Funds and in-kind support for its publication were provided by the Department of Veterans Affairs, the National Hospice and Palliative Care Organization, Ethos Consulting Group, LLC, and Rallying Points.

Thanks to staff at the following facilities, which hosted site visits: Bay Pines VAMC, St. Petersburg, Fla.; Hospice of St. Francis, Titusville, Fla.; the Hospice of the Florida Suncoast, Largo; Orlando (Fla.) VA Health Center; Tampa (Fla.) VA Health Center; and VA Palo Alto (Calif.) Health Care System; and to the veterans and their families at those facilities who shared their stories for this report. Author: Larry Beresford (510/536-3048; larryberesford@hotmail.com).

CHAPTER 9

Results of My Nonscientific, Revealing Survey

Over the years of my practice, I have traveled to many places and talked to many people. It seemed that just about everywhere I went, I met people with stories about their experiences with end-of-life care. Sometimes they were family members of someone who had died. Sometimes they were nurses. Sometimes they were physicians. Their stories were often moving, filled with questions and frustration, and some of them were really quite angry recollections of an unpleasant dying process.

As I was starting this book, I began to remember the power of those stories, and decided to create a Web site where people could share them. I created questionnaires appropriate for families, physicians, nurses, clergy, business and political leaders, and hospital administrators. The intention was to help each group focus upon the difficult problems presented by end-of-life care in America. These thoughts and ideas can contribute to our national dialogue so that we can begin to address the problems in our healthcare system regarding end-of-life care.

After some sections are a few comments from the Web site. Keep in mind this is not a scientific survey, but the thoughts and opinions are valid and reflect the feelings and comments I have encountered over the years.

FAMILIES

1. Most responders (two-thirds) said their physician had not discussed with the family that the dying process had begun and the concept of hospice had not been mentioned.
2. Few believed that they received a realistic appraisal of the situation.
3. Most responded that in retrospect, medical care during the dying process did not improve the situation.
4. Most of those responding did not have an advance directive. Among those who did, most did not find it to be helpful in their situation.

Selected comments:

- "A more realistic appraisal of outcome from the doctor and less pie-in-the-sky fantasy of recovery."
- "Hospice was wonderful to our family, and our doctor was very helpful in connecting us to hospice."

PHYSICIANS

1. More than half of the physician respondents said that legal concerns have influenced decisions in end-of-life care, causing prolongation of the dying process.
2. Many physicians responded that they present all possible options to their patient/family—including those they believe will benefit the patient, as well as those they believe will have no benefit or value, like putting a patient in the Intensive Care Unit.
3. Most physicians responded that their medical societies do not address the quality of end-of-life care.
4. Two-thirds believe medical societies should educate the public about the meaning of the permanent irreversible loss of the cerebral cortex, and it would be helpful to add this to the criteria of death.
5. Two-thirds of the physicians who filled out the survey believe the physician community has a responsibility to our society to use healthcare resources wisely. The overwhelming majority believes that this is not now the case.
6. A majority of physicians responding thought that *autonomy* means "Patients have the right to refuse appropriate care; no physician should offer, and no patient/family can demand, inappropriate care." They also believe that appropriate care is beneficial, supported by the best available medical evidence taking into account the patient's overall health and age. However, a majority of these physicians believe that over the years, consumerism and the possibility of legal action has caused them to provide nonbeneficial care and that a local panel of physicians, nurses, clergy, and a public representative should be available for support in difficult situations and to help unify a standard of care.
7. Most physicians agreed that healthcare costs in America are pricing many of our goods out of the global market, and physicians have a responsibility to make the wisest and best use of medical resources and treatment that bring the most beneficial care for the dollars spent.
8. By a two-to-one majority, responding physicians believe that hospitals encourage them to use billable technology, even when it may not be necessary.
9. About half answering the survey thought end-of-life care is becoming more aggressive (more attempts at cure and less palliative care), inhibiting referral to hospice.

Selected comments:

- "Physicians need an oversight resource like an appropriate care committee of physicians, nurses, clergy and a public representative available for support in difficult situations to help unify standards of care, and to provide guidance and support that would enhance the delivery of appropriate end-of-life care. Such a resource should be used carefully and thoughtfully."
- "Medical care is a fraud. I would [rather] fight in Iraq without a helmet than be in a U.S. hospital as a patient."
- "[I] dare not refuse care if family wants [it]."

NURSES

1. Two-thirds of the nurses responding to the survey have seen the dying process prolonged by nonbeneficial medical care. In addition, and almost all said that at least 50 percent of doctors do not know when to switch to palliative care and, over the past twenty years, are increasingly unable to stand up to families requesting/demanding useless care.
2. By a margin of two to one, the participants believe medical consumerism in end-of-life situations causes no benefit, but great expense. Almost half believe the hospital encourages high-tech over palliative care, even in end-of-life situations.
3. Two out of three nurses responding to the survey have seen patients entering the hospital from nursing homes when they should be in hospice.
4. A large majority of respondents are aware of a severe nursing shortage in the United States and believe that two-year hospital-based programs would enhance matriculation into nursing careers. Further, if hospitals offered further training to obtain a baccalaureate degree, many if not most of the two-year graduates would take advantage of that opportunity.
5. Three out of four of those participating in the survey agree that hospice is superior to nursing homes or hospitals for end-of-life situations, but that doctors are increasingly reluctant to declare that the dying process has begun because they are hesitant to commit to allowing the patient to die and instead of doing whatever the family wants.
6. Two out of three nurses responding believe that nonbeneficial end-of-life care is an economic barrier to universal coverage, and about half would be willing to serve on an appropriate care committee.

Selected comments:

- "It is difficult for many physicians to speak about hospice; to them it is thought to mean hopeless."

- "I think educating the public is paramount to overcoming the excessive waste of medical resources."
- "We need geriatric centers; [and a] big push for hospice awareness."
- "We need to scale down neonatal units' care."

CLERGY

1. Four out of five of the clergy participating in the survey believe most physicians do not have the necessary skills to recognize when it is proper to switch from curative to palliative care, nor do physicians refer patients to hospice in a timely manner.
2. About half of these clergy participants agree that permanent loss of the cerebral cortex should be additional criteria for death.
3. More than a third of the respondents would be willing to serve on an appropriate care committee.

Selected comments:

- "Be frank and honest with family when it is time to let go."
- "Doctors should be able to let go . . . I hope there is no money agenda in not referring patients [to hospice]."
- "I pray your work will reach a large audience and your findings will stimulate national dialogue."
- "[We need] honest discussion about what outcomes can be realistically expected in each case."
- "[We need] better training at medical school level."
- "[We need] family education to relieve guilt at ending active treatment."
- "[We need] education or chaplain involvement to show that hospice does not mean the doctor failed."
- "Religious leaders need to educate congregations on end-of-life issues."

HOSPITAL ADMINISTRATORS

The response from hospital administrators were too few and received mostly from outside of the United States to give any sense of hospital administrators' points of view.

BUSINESS LEADERS

1. Business leaders who answered the survey are concerned about our healthcare costs as they affect our global competitiveness. They agreed that our style of end-of-life care contributes significantly to those costs.
2. Almost unanimously, business leaders responding to the survey believe that our society is not getting value for its healthcare dollars, and that part of the reason is that hospitals do not use resources wisely.

3. Most business leaders responding thought if our percentage of gross domestic product devoted to healthcare were to decrease to that of Canada's, they would increase their workforces by at least 5 percent.

Options preferred by business leaders:

- Review hospital costs, especially nonbeneficial procedural fees and outliers.
- In the last three months of life insurance carriers pay 100 percent for hospice, but only 50 percent for nonhospice care.

POLITICAL LEADERS

1. Almost unanimously, those leaders responding to the survey thought our medical system does not deliver excellent end-of-life care. They cite the following reasons:
   - Too-frequent use of technology.
   - Inappropriate use of hospital facilities.
   - A protracted dying process.
   - Lack of physician skill.
2. Overwhelmingly, the political leaders who responded believe that the public is dissatisfied with our present medical system because of inappropriate use of hospital facilities and a lack of physician skills.
3. Political leaders responding to the survey thought that the reasons for problems with end-of-life care are a preoccupation with technology. They feel that those in charge of the healthcare system believe they need to use technology to remain financially viable.
4. They also feel that hospice use is inadequate.

CONCLUSION

It is unlikely we can improve our healthcare system without first determining the major problems in it, especially end-of-life care. I believe that surveys like these are the beginning of a constructive dialogue on the problems with the healthcare system of the United States, and end-of-life care in particular.

CHAPTER 10

The Winds of Change: Suggestions for New Directions in End-of-Life Care

Our dysfunctional end-of-life care is a product of our health system itself, and at the same time, serves as a mirror for the entire system. Many of the causes of our poorly functioning healthcare system originated in the unforeseen consequences of seemingly well-intentioned governmental action. Unfortunately, those unforeseen consequences have yet to be addressed.

Primary care physicians are the linchpin of any medical system. However, Medicare/Medicaid reimbursements for this specialty are grossly inadequate because of the large amount of funding devoted to procedures and the physicians who perform them.[1] This lack of adequate funding means fewer doctors enter the field, patients lose out on health education and preventive care, there is a lack of continuity of care, patients lose trust in the medical community, and many patients don't receive treatment until much later in the course of their disease.

Inadequate payment by Medicare/Medicaid for regular hospital bed care has many negative consequences. It encourages hospitals to promote intensive care and inappropriate use of technology and procedures to keep the institutions financially viable. It also encourages excessive use of technology and testing for patients who use the emergency room as their primary source of medical care.

Many nursing homes are on the verge of bankruptcy and are understaffed thanks to inadequate Medicaid funding and restrictive legal framework.[2] Because of this lack of funds and a host of arcane regulations, many nursing homes promote inappropriate referrals to acute care hospitals to take advantage of the Medicare benefit when the patient is referred back to the nursing home. This practices helps cover their reimbursement shortfalls between Medicare and Medicaid.[3] In my 40-plus years of hospital practice, I have seen this over and over again. I have seen the same patients, most with severe dementia, being admitted to the hospital, staying the time allowed by Medicare, then returned to the nursing home, only to be returned again when the Medicare/Medicaid time limits for nursing home care were nearing the maximum. These patients were totally unaware of who or where they were, they were often suffering, and most, if not all, should have been in hospice. Because there is no system to identify end-of-life patients and refer them to hospice within the nursing home, these patients are especially vulnerable to being shuttled back and forth between the nursing home and an acute care hospital. This creates misery for the patient and family, and is a tremendous waste of resources.

Because of the enormous expense of our overly procedural style of medicine, Medicare has decreased its funding for graduate medical education. Thus doctors in training have less time to assimilate the intricacies and complexities of medicine, and to develop the judgment necessary to use modern medicine appropriately. The physicians teaching our young doctors have less time to teach because they are required to generate funds by increasing their own patient loads. Hospitals' concern for bottom-line performance has driven medical education into directions that are not in the patients' best interests or the nation's best interest. Inappropriate end-of-life care is just one of those directions.

When Congress wrote the Patient Self-Determination Act (PSDA) and the Americans with Disabilities Act (ADA) without the caveat of what is medically appropriate for the patient, they failed to create a legal framework for appropriate end-of-life care. So misinterpretations of patient autonomy are not surprising. No wonder we have a misplaced sense of consumerism, disenchantment of the medical team, and a tremendous waste of resources. Congress has not adopted Medicare regulations that would allow on-site review by senior physicians in hospitals, nursing homes, and home care. This prevents the development of acceptable medical standards tailored to the individual case and encourages the use of costly inappropriate care.

Congress has also pandered to different special interests and lobbying groups, squandering an opportunity to inform the public about the permanent vegetative state through public expert medical testimony when controversy occurs. Congress's vulnerability to lobbying and special-interest groups has led to special consideration and funding for questionable practices by large drug and device-manufacturing corporations. A classic example is drug and device company financing physician research of their products or seeking physician endorsement of their products. In the case of drugs, the products being touted may be similar to or no more effective than products already on the market.[4] In the realm of devices, the cardiac stent has proven no more effective in stable coronary artery disease than standard medical therapy.[5] Yet it has become one of the most overused devices because device manufacturers push it, and Medicare will pay for it.

IS SINGLE PAYER THE ANSWER?

Medicare has not addressed alternatives to a single-payer system or come up with any alternatives that could save considerably on administrative expenses and facilitate a national electronic medical record system. Congress also has not created a method for revealing to working Americans their total payment into our healthcare system in the same way that they are informed of their Social Security contributions, as required by law.

Though almost all agree that every American needs health insurance, there are many objections expressed to the idea of national health insurance.[6] But we can distinguish between the financing of a system and how it operates. For example, public money could be used to buy private insurance for those who are not covered by insurance. Massachusetts has such a system. However, if our present practice of medicine continues unabated, the needed public monies will add to the already excessive portion of gross domestic product devoted to healthcare, causing an even greater distortion of our economy.

It is doubtful that a single central agency can determine the best health plan for all Americans and be able to deliver the ideal. If a single agency like the government determines distribution of revenue to all sectors of the healthcare system, the lobbying by each sector will become more intense than it is today. If Congress is in charge of our total healthcare system, the influence of lobbyists for the drug and device manufacturers, hospitals, and other special-interest groups will increase, not decrease.

With a centralized system, individuals and families would have a smaller voice in what is most appropriate for them, and no leverage over the institutions that affect their health. Individual choice would be lost in the system, especially as costs continue to increase, and congressional attempts at cost control become clumsy and arbitrary. Once the private health insurance industry is dismantled, it would be difficult to reconstruct it if a single payer system did not live up to expectations. A single-payer system for a nation of 300 million would be so large and so bureaucratic that innovation and adaptation to change would be extremely difficult.

Here's the big flaw in discussions of a single payer system at this time. Healthcare costs are now about 17 percent of GDP and already negatively affecting our national economy. Many companies cannot meet the cost of employee healthcare so either reduce their workforce dramatically, outsource labor overseas, or shut down altogether. The employee share of health insurance premiums continues to rise as well. The high cost of healthcare is definitely inhibiting the ability of many companies to grow, and it could get worse unless there is significant change. The U.S. Government Accounting Office projects that by 2075, a full one-fifth of GDP will be devoted to federal spending for just Medicare, Medicaid, and Social Security.[7] Numbers like that could bankrupt the economy.

If we add even more money to the system without fixing the problems first, it could have an even greater negative impact on the economic situation. We know that the sense of well-being of our citizens often reflects the health of our economy. Therefore, one might conclude that if the economy deteriorates further, so might the health and well-being of the American people.

In a global economy, if one nation has to increase its price for goods and services because of an overly expensive healthcare system, its competitiveness is compromised and so is its economy. No matter how the financing of our healthcare is eventually worked out, we must deal with the excessive costs of our present system. A big part of this cost is inappropriate care of our citizens at the end of their lives.

Yet another author supports this view and contends that the present system is designed to serve the economic, professional, and political interests of physicians, hospitals, and drug and insurance companies—and not the health of our citizens.[8] We need a system that cares for the uninsured, provides evidence-based medicine that gives real value for healthcare dollars, promotes the corner stone of primary care, and provides care tailored to the unique needs of each patient, especially at the end of life.

PROPOSALS FOR CHANGE: SOLUTIONS ARE BORN OUT OF PROBLEMS

I have already discussed some of the solutions in greater detail in previous chapters. Here is a short version of each one, along with a few other solutions that I have not previously covered in detail. If even just one or two of them became reality, it would make a difference in how patients are treated at the end of their lives. My goal, however, is to see a huge groundswell of support for meaningful and far-ranging change. That means let's go for all of them!

Address the Unintended Consequences of the PSDA and the ADA

Congress must amend the PSDA and ADA and add a clause to both that reads: "Every patient has the right to evidence-based care tailored to the individual, but cannot choose care that is deemed nonbeneficial by the weight of medical evidence and the patients' overall health. Local, state and national appropriate care committees will be available to adjudicate any disagreements. Patients of sound mind and of legal age have the right to refuse any or all appropriate care."

To address problems specific to the PSDA, Congress should add the following clause: "Patients of sound mind and of legal age may refuse any or all therapy where the expected benefits significantly outweigh the possible complications."

To remedy problems resulting from the ADA, Congress should add the following clause: "Patients with disabilities should receive appropriate care when the expected benefits significantly outweigh the possible complications."

These amendments are meant for those cases in which there is no doubt that a particular therapy will not benefit the patient. This congressional action would send a loud and clear message that medical science and knowledge are important factors that must take priority in medical decisions.

Change Outdated CPR Policy

The CPR by default policy, developed in the 1960s, is no longer appropriate as the hospital patient population continues to age. It is not only an often useless procedure in end-of-life cases, but it can also cause great suffering for the patient. CPR should only be performed after an assessment of the overall condition of the patient shows that it will benefit the patient in the long run. The American Heart

Association/International Liaison Committee on Resuscitation should address this issue at their next guideline meeting in 2010, and change the CPR by default status to CPR in appropriate situations only. Doing away with CPR by default could also save billions of dollars in needless and hopeless end-of-life treatment.

Create a New Style of Hospital Admission Form

As you learned in Chapter 2, the PSDA and the promotion of advance directives have created countless nightmares for end-of-life patients and their families.

Instituting changes to the PSDA and ADA, developing a new policy on CPR, and creating appropriate care committees would go a long way toward keeping cases out of the courts, where decisions about patient care are often based more on legal precedent than sound medical and scientific data.

My proposal for a new style of hospital admission form (Figure 10.1) would essentially create an advance directive that is fresh and timely with each hospital admission. It would eliminate many of the questions about what a patient might want in the absence of an advance directive, relieve families and physicians of the burden of deciding if a do not resuscitate (DNR) order is needed, designate CPR status on the form, and ensure that the patient receives appropriate care.

Establish an Appropriate Care Committee System

Chapter 3 clearly makes the case for Appropriate Care Committees. Even though most hospitals have an ethics committee, they simply don't have the clout to do much more than make recommendations. A structured, three-tiered system (local, state, and national) of Appropriate Care Committees like the ones I have suggested would support the ethics committees, but have more power to ensure that beneficial care is delivered to all patients, especially those at the end of their lives. They would have the authority to withhold payment for care deemed inappropriate. They would be paid a stipend, therefore their decisions would not be influenced by any financial considerations, and would be based solely on the appropriateness of care.

Bring Primary Care Back to the Forefront

The advent of Medicare/Medicaid, and the expansion of insurance companies' procedure-based payment system, have essentially devalued primary care. Consequently, over the past 40 years the brightest and best have pursued emergency medicine, radiology, dermatology, and the surgical or medical subspecialties, rather than seeking a career as primary care physician. As the influence of subspecialists has grown, the prestige and earning power of the primary care physician has decreased. We see many primary care physicians struggling to earn a living, while those who have chosen the world of procedural medicine are earning colossal incomes.

Figure 10.1. Proposed Admission Form.

Patient Name _____
Med. Record # _____
D.O.B. _____
Date _____

Is Patient capable of decision making {yes ( ) No ( )}; if not who is
responsible?_____

**A patient has the right to evidence based care tailored to the individual, but
cannot receive care that has no value. The physician team is responsible for
defining beneficial care, where the benefit to the patient significantly exceeds the
risks. A committee (the appropriate care committee) is available within the
hospital should conflict arise. The committee will render judgment within one
working day.**

Cardiopulmonary Resuscitation (CPR) is ordered on this patient

Yes ( )   No ( )

**The patient/family has placed the following restrictions on CPR because
of personal choice even though it is medically indicated. DO NOT DO
THE FOLLOWING**

( ) intubation   ( ) chest compression   ( ) resuscitation drugs   ( ) cardioversion

**Other therapies this patient has chosen to refuse even though medically
indicated are:**

_____
_____
_____
_____

**When thought to be in an end of life situation by the medical team, I want to
receive palliative care and consider placement in Hospice**

Yes ( )   No ( )

The appropriate care I want is:

_____

Physician Signature _____

Patient Signature _____

Witness Signature _____

Source: © Copyright 2007, Kenneth A. Fisher, M.D.

Now we have an absolutely absurd situation. Primary care physicians must see
thirty to forty patients per day to make a modest living. Instead of spending a
minimum of 30 minutes with each patient and being reimbursed a reasonable
amount, the primary care physician is spending approximately 12–15 minutes per
patient. As Dr. Brown pointed out in the Foreword, how can a physician possibly

get to know even a few of the myriad factors that play into a patient's condition? How can questions be asked and answered, concerns be addressed, or a deep trusting relationship between doctor and patient be nurtured when the doctor is so rushed he or she has to get down to the nitty-gritty, then get on to the next patient?

When physicians have to see patients at this rapid rate, they are physically and emotionally exhausted, and they are mentally spent by the end of the day. No wonder burnout is near epidemic proportions among primary care physicians. The hectic, crazy-making schedules and compromised incomes are no secret in the halls of the medical schools. As a result, the lure of young doctors toward primary care, a life "in the trenches" serving local communities, is bordering upon extinction.

In order to maintain the caseload, primary care physicians can't really afford to leave the office to see their patients that are in the hospital. That has to be left to the "hospitalist," or general internist who practices only in the hospital, taking care of other physicians' patients. Patients are asked to trust a physician they have never seen before and, in most hospitals, multiple hospitalists during a single admission. Primary care doctors, whom the patients have known for years and come to trust, do not interact with their patients during the hospital admission.

Now here's another twist that enters into the picture. During the same time period that hospitals began to generate funds in earnest for growth and new building, a push to discharge patients as soon as possible also began. The result has been a new area of internal medicine. Hospitalists become very adept at caring for these sicker patients, who may require more procedures, so are usually able to discharge other patients in a shorter period of time, even if another day or so in the hospital might be beneficial. This is one of the mechanisms at work in the shift away from a more personal approach to medicine to the procedure-based style of medicine that generates the most money. As all this has evolved, the primary care physician has watched the funds flow away.

Procedures at the right time for the right patient are appropriate, but we have gone far beyond what is appropriate in many cases. Here's where Appropriate Care Committees come in. As they review cases, and reduce the number of inappropriate procedures, the Medicare/Medicaid funds that are saved could be channeled to the primary care physicians. We would be able to compensate primary care physicians at a rate that would allow them to visit with a patient for a minimum of 30 minutes. With adequate compensation, the primary physicians would be able leave the office to go see their patients who are in the hospital at least once during the hospital stay and insist that the hospitalist keep them updated daily on patient status. This human contact with the primary care physician would go a long way in satisfying our society's dissatisfaction with our medical system.

Prepare the Medical Community to Deal with the Growing Population of Frail Elderly

There's no question that the number of frail elderly patients entering medical and nursing facilities will increase dramatically in the very near future. The big question is: Will the medical community make the drastic changes necessary to create a system that provides superior care for our seniors without putting our country into bankruptcy?

Institutional care, nursing homes, and acute care hospitals cannot be the mainstay of the care for this population. Institutional care is not only impersonal, it is far too expensive for this purpose. Treatment in an acute care facility is certainly appropriate when it is needed, but the mainstay of care will have to be a noninstitutional setting, preferably at home. This would translate into a robust home care capability. Teams led by physicians would include visiting nurses, nurse's aides, and homemakers, all skilled in caring for elderly and frail patient in a home setting.

We cannot underestimate the importance of physician judgment in directing a home care program. Physicians will have to be experts in palliative and hospice care, and use that expertise to make decisions, to ask patients and families the right questions, and to be prepared to answer the questions and concerns of those same patients and families. Physicians will also have to be skilled in leading the home care teams, with the primary goal of tailoring and coordinating the best possible services for each patient. Primary care and geriatric programs in medical schools will have to revamp their training to be sure that graduates have these special skills.

Can we, as a nation, afford to provide this type of care? The larger question is: can we afford *not* to? We can no longer afford our present model of putting most of the frail elderly in institutions. It is not only an outrageous squandering of resources, it also perpetuates an impersonal system of medicine that dishonors the role of touch and compassion in end-of-life care.

Reverse the Nursing Shortage

It is unethical for our country to be luring nurses from other countries to meet our nursing needs when their native countries desperately need them at home. At the same time, we certainly need to reverse the nursing shortage very soon to meet the demands of a mushrooming elderly population. Nurses are the mainstays of care in hospitals and nursing homes and will be crucial to the success of physician-led palliative care teams of the future.

The U.S. Health Resources and Services Administration has suggested raising nursing salaries to match other comparable careers to lure nurses back into the profession, recruiting and graduating more nurses from college-level nursing programs, and encouraging nurses to work beyond normal retirement age. They also suggest that changes in Social Security retirement ages may influence retirement plans for many nurses.[9]

As I discussed in Chapter 5, I would add to this list the return of the two-year, in-hospital training programs that declined, then vanished as more emphasis was placed on university training for nurses. These programs turned out excellent nurses and offered opportunities to many people who might not otherwise have afforded them. The same is just as true now, especially in our cities. There is a rich pool of bright, talented people who might well choose nursing as a career if a financially realistic option was available. The federal government, through Medicare and other means, has a long history of stimulating education to increase the number of healthcare professionals. A similar inducement could be initiated for nursing education. This would make it profitable for hospitals to reenter the area of nursing education and I feel that many, if not most, would initiate these programs.

Redefine Death to Include Loss of the Cerebral Cortex

In Chapter 1, I reviewed the 1968 origins of the definition of brain death, a definition that when carefully considered is in frank contradiction with reality. In Chapter 4, I discussed how this definition has created a huge dilemma for families with loved ones in the persistent vegetative state. While it is true that some patients may recover to varying degrees, many will not. A quite simple test to determine complete and irrevocable loss of the cerebral cortex would be the blood flow scan of the head that shows no blood flow to that part of the brain. The American Academy of Neurology could amend or add to this determination. This test would remove questions about the potential for recovery.

Some theorize it would be easier to maintain the old definition of brain death rather than redefine brain death to include permanent loss of the cerebral cortex, but *treat* loss of the cerebral cortex as if it is equivalent to total brain death. However, such a strategy also implies that physicians, nurses, and the public already understand that it is equivalent to brain death and might find it appropriate to cease all therapy. In a litigious society such as ours this reference could be wrought with pitfalls.

The American Academy of Neurology must expressly add irrevocable loss of the cerebral cortex as an additional definition of death, and specify how that irrevocable loss is to be determined. Certainly many would object, and such a move would inspire vigorous medical, scientific, and ethical debate. That in itself would be a good thing and would bring critical questions at the core of this fundamental issue of life and death into the light. Traditionalists might argue that for millennia cessation of respiratory or cardiac function have been the definitions of death. But back then there were no respiratory ventilators, pacemakers, feeding tubes, antibiotics, Foley catheters, IV fluids, and all the other technologies of modern medicine.

The numbers of people in the United States in persistent vegetative states is unknown, since there have been no definitive studies. Estimates range from 10 thousand to 40 thousand, depending on what study you read. Of those, there are no statistics on how many actually have total and irreversible loss of the cerebral cortex based on a definitive test. However, a conservative estimate of the cost of caring for such a patient is around $50,000 a year. If only 10 thousand of those patients were without cerebral cortical function, that translates into $500 million a year in futile care. But more important is the human cost. The families must carry the memory of a person who can never return, endure a mourning period that seemingly never ends, and hope for a recovery that never comes.

Reduce the Cost of Healthcare Administration

Twenty percent of the $2 trillion yearly healthcare expenditure is for administrative expenses. That's $400 *billion*! Just too much money. There are armies of billers working for healthcare facilities, pitted against another army of bureaucrats working for the insurance companies who often reject claims based only on administrative data, rather than individual patient circumstances. Every private insurance policy has its specific coverages, and insurance companies scrutinize every bill to be sure it is only paying for what is covered. Meanwhile, every healthcare facility tries to maximize its bill by following the intricacies of the patient's insurance company.

Medicare uses a completely different approach. The Medicare billing codes contain thousands of pages of contradicting rules. If, for some reason a healthcare facility should be reviewed, Medicare could always find it in violation of one rule or another. So the providing facility needs yet another army of billers to keep up with what Medicare is looking for at any particular period of time.

How do we fix this waste of energy, manpower, and money? Some advise doing away with private insurers, and let everything be Medicare. If that were to be the case, instead of thousands of pages of code, Medicare could generate *hundreds* of thousands of pages of code. Better not run afoul of its computer. You could be long dead before the problem would be fixed.

You probably don't know this, but the Medicare payment system is a contractual relationship between the federal government and various private insurers in different regions of the country. Might it be possible to develop a single billing system, not a single-payer system?

Congress could create an independent agency like the Federal Reserve Bank that would essentially be a "Healthcare Bank." All insurance companies would pay that "bank." All healthcare facilities would bill and receive their funds from that "bank." A portion of all insurers' funds, to be determined by the "bank," would be allocated to medical research through the National Institutes of Health, as would an amount for graduate medical education. Thus, a fraction of all insurers' funds would be dedicated to the future of medicine, in proportion to the percentage of the population covered by them. The "bank" would also fund the Appropriate Care Committee system, and would be off-limits to lobbying by special-interest groups like drug and medical device companies.

All insurance companies and federal and state governments would have a fixed number of insurance packages or coverages for their clients. The various computer information technology companies would write programs so that each facility could interface with the central computer system run by the "bank."

There would still be plenty of opportunity for each insurance company to innovate around the fixed number of packages. Packages would be reviewed and adjusted for a changing world every two years. The "bank" would then be a depository for every admitting history and physical and discharge summary. An elaborate privacy system that is HIPAA-compliant would ensure that only authorized individuals, like the patient's physician(s), would have access to the records to maintain security of personal information. Also, the information technology companies would write compatibility programs so that only appropriate, authorized individuals would have access to the individual patient's hospital computer system giving access to retrieve all laboratory and X-ray data.

A system like this would have a good chance of cutting our administrative costs in half. That alone would save our nation about $200 billion every year, and would be much less confusing for patients, physicians, and facility administrators. The savings could be channeled into nursing education, primary care, and expanding palliative care and hospice services.

Reform Drug Company and Medical Device Advertising

Direct-to-consumer advertising by drug companies greatly expanded in the mid-1990s because of changes in Food and Drug Administration (FDA) rules and regulations.[10] A 2007 study published in the *New England Journal of Medicine* found drug company advertising increased from $11.4 billion in 1996 to $29.9 billion in 2005.[11] In 2005, 14 percent of that $29.9 billion was spend to direct-to-consumer advertising. That's over $4 billion! This does not include drug company support for patient groups and charitable organizations that can advertise without reporting their sources to the FDA. In 2004, all major drug companies but two spent more than twice as much on marketing/advertising and administration than on research.[12]

The marketing promises results out of proportion to reality and helps create the image that magical cures are just a pill away. The marketing of newer, more expensive drugs of the same class as older, cheaper drugs with proven safety records is also troublesome. The marketing efforts make medicine seem simple. If you have this problem, take this drug. This kind of advertising glosses over the potential risk versus potential gain and ignores entirely the fact that each case is different and complex. The ads help create the impression that there is a drug for every problem, and that more drugs means better care.

The ads also perpetuate the myth that the American consumer may be paying more than any other nation for drugs, but that the extra expense is worth it because it funds much-needed research. Actually, what it funds is profit levels that are higher than any other industry, bringing in profits more than five times the average of the Fortune 500.[13] In reality, the American consumer is taking too many drugs, and paying too much for each one of them.

Drug company sponsorship of research by academic institutions is another area of concern. Pharmaceutical companies frequently sponsor studies to demonstrate that their drug is superior to the older, cheaper drugs of the same class already on the market. However, if studies do not go their way, they will prohibit them from being published and can be quite aggressive in doing so.[14] In 2002, the FDA approved 78 new drugs, with only seven classified as significant improvements on older drugs. Not a single one of the seven classified as drugs of improvement were developed by a major U.S. drug company.

The pharmaceutical industry is not alone in marketing for bigger profits. The medical device industry, particularly for cardiovascular, orthopedic, and eye disorders, is now a $400 billion industry.[15] Here there is the same concern that physicians conducting the studies that prove the efficacy of devices are unduly influenced by the company. While there have been conferences devoted to this difficult issue, no satisfactory solutions have emerged.[16] I propose that all clinical trials by drug and device companies be funded through the NIH to ensure that the best possible research design and data analysis are being performed.

The general course for devices is that they are approved by Medicare and other insurers for specific circumstances and indications. There is no doubt that the benefits outweigh the risks for patients with these indications. However, there is the temptation to expand their use through ads to the public, to the financial advantage of both the industry and physicians who prescribe them. The insurance carriers pay for the procedure regardless of any proven benefit for a particular patient. Frequently, after many years of unproven application and tens of billions of dollars in payments, a clinical study is finally performed that debunks the expanded use of the device. The classic example is the overuse of coronary artery stents.[17]

How do we remedy this situation? One suggestion would be to return to the prohibition of direct-to-consumer advertising by the pharmaceutical and medical device industries. Whatever the reasons for removing the ban of direct to consumer advertising for prescription drugs in the 1990s, that action in retrospect was a huge error and should be rescinded. Another suggestion is to instruct the FDA to stop certifying "me-too" drugs, thus encouraging the pharmaceutical industry to use their research dollars on creative new solutions to our multiple healthcare problems like cocaine and heroin addiction, violent behavior, and obesity.*

Increase and Redirect Funding for Medical Education

As I discussed in earlier chapters, Medicare funding for medical education has decreased over the past 10 years. That has created such problems as not enough time to study and learn, and physicians not having enough time to teach because of the emphasis on increasing patient load to generate more funds for the hospital. Not only are the physicians-in-training not getting the education they deserve, our society also suffers when their training does not emphasize humanness and caring. These trainees are the future physicians of America. It is not in the national interest for our future physicians to be trained this way.

A second problem is that the funding of residency and fellowship programs that provide further training beyond residency in a specific specialty—like cardiology, gastroenterology, or oncology—flows through the hospitals. Thus, hospital administrators control physician training through control of the funding. Almost all hospital administrators scrupulously protect the actual amount of money they receive for resident and fellow training that may amount to hundreds of millions of dollars. The actual amount is often a mystery. Hospitals may have to spend more on their residents and fellows, but these trainees provide many hours of

---

*(To read more, see Appendix 6: Surviving Sepsis—Practice Guidelines, Marketing Campaigns, and Eli Lilly.)

availability and around-the-clock patient services. It would cost a hospital a small fortune if they had to be replaced with practicing physicians.

We need a goal-oriented policy—a policy that allows residents and fellows to learn their craft and become knowledgeable, kind, humane doctors. It takes time for trainees to master analytical thinking and complex problem solving, acquire necessary technical and procedure-based skills, and to reflect upon the social and psychological impact their new role has upon their patients and peers, and upon themselves as well. The hands-on guidance, as well as emotional support by experienced physicians and surgeons, is critical to the growth of the finest doctors.

The first step would be to remove the funds currently allotted toward graduate medical education to hospitals and create separate boards composed of educators and representatives of the medical community, who would receive and manage these funds. Graduate Medical education is a specific task that should receive its funding directly from third party payers and not through intermediaries like hospitals or medical schools.

With the present system of hospitals skimming money from education funds, it is impossible to judge if present-day funding is adequate. This would have to be carefully studied by the healthcare corporation described earlier in this chapter. Perhaps it would require more funds. However, if suggestions made in this chapter were to be adopted, the amount of money needed to enhance medical education would likely be minuscule compared to the money saved.

Medical Societies Must Speak Up

Many people, especially in the medical community, viewed the silence of the American Medical Association, the American College of Physicians, and the American Academy of Neurology during the national dialogue about the Terri Schiavo controversy as a dereliction of societal responsibility. It is the responsibility of the medical societies to educate the public about the realities of the persistent vegetative state and the permanent absence of a cerebral cortex and to willfully invite dialogue regarding this and other complex medical issues.

A primary objective of our medical societies should be the concept of physicians delivering value in healthcare. With the current calls for universal healthcare coverage, our expensive style of medicine will dramatically increase the percentage of gross domestic product devoted to healthcare. As the percentage of gross domestic product devoted to healthcare approaches 20 percent, this cost will negatively impact our economy. Congress will be forced to take action in the midst of a crisis. The chances of Congress creating a plan that would be excellent for physicians, medical facilities, patients, the insurance industry, and our society at large is close to slim and none. Drastic congressional action under duress will most likely inhibit physician ability to individualize our care of patients.

Medical societies should be at the forefront of examining our CPR policy, excessive ICU care, poor end-of-life care, inappropriate admissions of end-of-life nursing home patients to hospitals, excessive use of technology such as dialysis at the end of life, stents for stable angina, administration of chemotherapy when the likelihood of response is more a function of hope than chance of remission, and intrathoracic cardiac defibrillators, just to name a few. It strains for the credibility of our medical societies to work against physician reimbursement cuts and not look at the wasted resources caused by excessive technology and procedures for our patients at the same time.

If medical societies would rise to the challenge of addressing these quandaries, a drastic shift in the current medical culture and its paradigm would follow. They should be champions of appropriate care for our citizens. This transformation would not only ensure a new sense of value for the dollar for our society, but might fuel the novel experience of technology and humanism as complimentary rather than antagonistic.

Oversight and Review

The United States is a world leader in technological and procedural medicine. Acquisition and mastery of these skills are intrinsic to our leadership role in medical advancement. No doubt they will continue to be nurtured by our society and its social, political, and economic policies. The problem is not in the development of technology and procedures. It is in their application. The lack of oversight and consistent review of policies and procedures is largely what has gotten us in the mess we're in now.

There is one area where oversight is sadly lacking. Patients may be receiving more medication than they need at levels that may be unsafe, and insurance companies and Medicare/Medicaid continue to pay the enormous tab. A 2007 article in the *Journal of the American Medical Association* looked at the use of epoetin, a drug used for patients receiving dialysis, which is covered by Medicare. They found that epoetin use was much higher in for-profit hospitals and franchised dialysis chains (specialty hospitals), than in nonprofit hospitals. There is even some question as to whether technicians were encouraged to use higher dosages, especially in the large, for-profit chains, and whether those increases were warranted.[18]

Even if every single one of the recommendations in this chapter were implemented, it would be crucial that they be periodically and methodically reviewed for effectiveness, especially in the face of new or emerging healthcare issues. This will be most important as the elderly population booms, and end-of-life care is the near-dominant focus.

So there you have it. As I see it, the future of our healthcare system is in our hands, and if we all join together—healthcare people, businesspeople, politicians, and just plain folks—we can be a powerful force for meaningful change. And if we want change, we must act boldly and quickly. We cannot wait until the system is so bloated that we find ourselves in a major economic crisis, and the bureaucrats step in to create something that none of us will like very much at all.

We can do it. I'm game. Are you?

Appendix 1

The Survey Questionnaires

BUSINESS LEADERS SURVEY

1. Do you receive your medical care in the United States?
   Yes   No

2. Are you concerned about healthcare costs in the United States and our global competitiveness?
   Yes   No

3. Do you believe our present end-of-life style of care is a significant part of our healthcare costs?
   Yes   No

4. Why do you think our national healthcare costs, as a percentage of the gross domestic product, exceed any other nations? (Check all that apply.)

   — We as a nation use too many expensive drugs
   — Our hospitals do not use technologies wisely
   — Physicians have little or no concern regarding the use of resources
   — We emphasize technological versus humane care
   — Our national administrative costs are great
   — As long as others are paying our public does not mind "overusing" healthcare
   — Other

5. Do you believe our society is getting "value" for its healthcare dollars?
   Yes   No

6. What do you believe is the reason this issue is not being addressed nationally?

   — Inertia (fear of change)
   — Fear of interest groups

— Past failures
— An ambivalent public
— Thinks more is better
— Does not understand the impact on our national economics.
— Likes fancy new buildings
— Is confused about the Patient Self-Determination Act
— Other

7. If the United States were to decrease its percentage of gross domestic product for health care to that of Canada and other Western societies, your workforce would increase by what percentage?

— 1–5%
— 6–10%
— 11–20%
— 21% or more

8. What suggestions would you make to improve our healthcare system?

— Review hospital costs especially nonbeneficial procedural fees and outliers.
— Medicare pays in last three months of life 100% for hospice, 50% for non-hospice care.
— Congress mandates that insurance companies create a single "agency" to process all healthcare bills and create a national system for an electronic medical record. Goal is to get administrative costs to approach 5% from the present 20%.
— Comfort homes are created where care is given to maximize comfort vs. medical care in nursing homes as a stage between nursing homes and hospice.
— Congress advises states to refine criteria for death as loss of cerebral function.
— Medical societies have a responsibility to educate the public regarding what is a human without a functioning cerebral cortex.
— Congress clarifies the Personnel Self-Determination Act to develop procedures to ensure that patient autonomy means patients have the right to refuse appropriate care, but no physician should offer and no patient/family can demand inappropriate care based on best available medical evidence.
— The benefits to our society of having healthcare the same or slightly higher percentage of Gross Domestic Product as other Western countries
— Define what is appropriate criteria for various technologies
— Supply expert witnesses and legal support if these criteria are followed and legal action ensues.
— Take steps (i.e., regional committees) to help with standards of care.
— Other

9. Please feel free to make any other suggestions or comments regarding health-care policy.

CLERGY SURVEY

1. Do you receive your medical care in the United States?
Yes   No

2. About how many end-of-life situations do you minister to each year?

   — 0–10
   — 11–20
   — 21–50
   — 51–100
   — Greater than 100

3. Overall how would you rate our present medical systems' approach to end-of-life care?

   — Almost universally delivers effective end-of-life care
   — Frequently delivers effective end-of-life care
   — Rarely delivers effective end-of-life care
   — Does not understand what is effective end-of-life care

4. Do you believe most physicians have the necessary skill to recognize when it is time to switch from curative to palliative care?
Yes   No

5. In our healthcare system do you think hospice provides the best end-of-life care?
Yes   No

6. If so, do you think doctors refer patients to hospice in a timely manner?
Yes   No

7. What suggestions would you make to improve referral to hospice?

8. The human spirit, all consciousness, thinking, purposeful movement, speech, all activity we call human is seated in our cerebral cortex. Bodily functions, like respiration, are controlled by lower brain areas, i.e., brainstem. Would you consider permanent loss of brain cortical function as additional criteria for human death?
Yes   No

9. Please feel free to make any suggestions that you feel would improve our nation's end-of-life care.

10. Would you be willing to participate on a committee (with physicians, nurses and lay representation) that would help adjudicate difficult end-of-life situations and help with standards of care?
Yes   No

FAMILY SURVEY

1. Do you receive your medical care in the United States?
   Yes   No

2. Where did your family member or person you were caring for die? Check all appropriate answers.

   — Hospital
   — Hospice within hospital
   — Home with hospice
   — Home without hospice
   — Nursing home
   — Separate hospice facility
   — Other

3. During the last three months of life where did the dying person spend most of the time?

   — Hospital
   — Hospice within hospital,
   — Home with hospice
   — Home without hospice
   — Nursing home
   — Independent hospice facility
   — Other

4. In retrospect, do you think your family member had a prolonged death? (This would be a protracted course of dying, not an extension of quality living.)
   Yes   No

   If yes, for how long? (circle the most appropriate answer)
   Days   Weeks   Months   Years

5. Did the physician(s) ever discuss with you the possibility that the dying process had begun?
   Yes   No

   If yes, at what point? (Circle the most appropriate answer)
   After Days   After Weeks   After Months   After Years

6. Was the possibility of gospice ever mentioned?
   Yes   No

   If you answered yes, at what point? (Circle the most appropriate answer)
   After Days   After Weeks   After Months   After Years

7. Was your family member at some point in a hospital during this final episode?
   Yes   No

   If you answered yes, do you believe you received a realistic appraisal of the situation?
   Yes   No

If in the hospital at some point during this final episode, was there a phase in the Intensive Care Unit (ICU)?
Yes   No

If yes, do you believe the stay in the ICU was beneficial?
Yes   No

8. Did your family member at some point in the dying process lose the ability to reason?
Yes   No

If yes, at what time was this before death? (Circle the most appropriate answer)
Days Before   Weeks Before   Months Before   Years Before

9. Did the healthcare team encourage you or other family members to assume responsibility for making decisions regarding stopping life-extending therapy?
Yes   No

If yes, were some of the choices using high-technology care which in retrospect were useless?
Yes   No

10. If high technology was used which in retrospect was useless, for what period of time before death? (Circle the most appropriate answer)
Days Before   Weeks Before   Months Before   Years Before

11. Looking back, do you feel that during the dying process the medical care improved the process?
Yes   No

12. Do you believe the dying person had a lingering death?
Yes   No

If yes, for how long?
Days   Weeks   Months   Years

13. Did the dying person have an advance directive?
Yes   No

If yes, was it helpful?
Yes   No

14. If there was an advance directive, did the medical team follow it?
Yes   No

15. During what you would call the dying process was your family member readmitted to the hospital?
Yes   No

If you answered yes, how many times? (Circle the most appropriate answer)
Once   2–3   4–5   6 or more

If readmitted, do you believe the hospital stay was helpful?
Yes   No

16. Do you think this end-of-life episode cost:

    — Hundreds of dollars
    — Thousands of dollars
    — Tens of thousands of dollars
    — Hundreds of thousands of dollars
    — Millions of dollars

17. If you wish, please comment how in retrospect the dying process of your family member could have been improved.

18. Please use the space below to make any comments about your experience.

HOSPITAL ADMINISTRATION SURVEY

1. Do you receive your medical care in the United States?
   Yes   No

2. Do you think the U.S. healthcare system is too expensive while not providing care to all?
   Yes   No

3. Do you think that nonbeneficial care to the dying instead of hospice adds to this problem?
   Yes   No

4. Is your hospital affiliated with a hospice?
   Yes   No

5. Do you believe that an in-hospital hospice unit could provide a more comfortable and appropriate setting for the patients who die in your hospital?
   Yes   No

6. Do you have an in-hospital hospice in your hospital?
   Yes   No

   If no, what are the reasons?

7. Have you in the past ten years added ICU beds in your hospital?
   Yes   No

8. Approximately how many patients die in your ICU yearly?

    — 0–10
    — 11–20
    — 21–50
    — 51–100
    — Greater than 100

9. There is increasing evidence that advance directives are not working; do you agree?
   Yes   No

10. Is there an increasing problem of patients/families requesting (demanding) tests and treatments that physicians believe are not indicated?
    Yes   No

11. Have you found over the same period of time that physicians have become more reluctant to express their judgment as to what is appropriate care, and to prescribe palliative rather than curative care?
Yes   No

12. Do you believe that some of the patients that enter your hospital should have entered hospice instead?
Yes   No

If yes, why did they not enter hospice?

13. Do you believe that medical societies should provide more support for individual doctors especially when there is conflict with patients/families?
Yes   No

14. Have Medicare/Medicaid reimbursement policies caused you to decrease general floor nursing and increase intensive care beds?
Yes   No

15. What suggestions would you make to better care for dying patients in your hospital?

NURSES AND OTHER CARE GIVERS SURVEY

1. Do you receive your medical care in the United States?
Yes   No

2. Have you seen the dying process prolonged by nonbeneficial medical care?
Yes   No

If yes, about what percentage by doctors who do not know when to switch to palliative care?

— >75%
— 75%
— 50%
— 25%
— <25%

If yes, about what percentage by families insisting on more curative care and physicians who to avoid conflict and possible lawsuits go along?

— >75%
— 75%
— 50%
— 25%
— <25%

3. Does it appear to you that doctors have become less willing to use their judgment as to what is appropriate care over the past fifteen to twenty years?
Yes   No

4. Do you think that medical consumerism in end-of-life situations has reached a point where little is accomplished but at great expense?
Yes   No

5. Do you think that the facility that you work encourages high-tech care, even when palliative care would seem more reasonable for the patient at this point in time?
   Yes   No

6. Have you seen decreasing care capability on general wards with more patients going into Intensive Care Units?
   Yes   No

7. Have you seen patients from nursing homes enter your hospital when it would be more appropriate for them to be in hospice?
   Yes   No

8. Are you aware of a severe nursing shortage in the United States?
   Yes   No

9. If yes, do you think if hospitals reinstituted two-year programs more Americans than presently going into nursing school would enroll?
   Yes   No

10. If hospitals had additional programs so that the two-year graduates could obtain B.S. degrees would many (if not most) take advantage of that program?
    Yes   No

11. Do you believe that hospice is better for dying patients than a hospital or a nursing home?
    Yes   No

12. Do you believe that doctors are increasingly reluctant to declare that the dying process has begun?
    Yes   No

    If yes is this because (check all that apply)

    — They no longer have the skills
    — They are reluctant to commit
    — They do pretty much what the patient/family wants
    — Other

13. Our healthcare system is extremely expensive and yet we have many millions uninsured. Do you think nonbeneficial medical care of the dying significantly adds to this problem?
    Yes   No

14. Would you be willing to serve on a local committee with two physicians, clergy, and lay representatives sponsored by medical and nursing societies to help adjudicate end-of-life standards of care?
    Yes   No

Please feel free to make further suggestions or comments.

PHYSICIAN SURVEY

1. Do you receive your medical care in the United States?
   Yes   No

2. During your career, have you provided end-of-life care?
Yes   No
If yes, approximately how many patients?
— 1–9
— 10–40
— 50–99
— 100–999
— 1,000 or more

3. Have legal issues ever influenced you in your approach to these cases?
Yes   No

If yes:
— A few
— Many
— Most
— All

4. If yes, in your opinion has your consideration of legal issues led to the prolongation of the dying process?
Yes   No

If yes, for how long? (Circle the most appropriate answer)
Days   Weeks   Months   Years

5. In discussion of options with dying patients, with the patient/family/guardian, do you usually present:

— All possible options (including those you think will not result in improving/extending the quality of the patient's life)
— Only options which you think will improve the quality of the patient's life.
— Options that use technology, whether or not they improve the quality of the patient's life.
— Hospice.
— Other.

6. Have you put patients in an Intensive Care Unit while thinking there was little or no chance of improvement?
Yes   No

If yes:
— On rare occasions
— Some of the time
— Most of the time
— Always

7. Has any medical society in your state or nationally brought to your attention the quality of end-of-life care in your area?
Yes   No

If yes, has this involved?
— Physician-assisted suicide

— Alleviation of pain and suffering
— Appropriate use of resources
— Hospice
— Legal issues
— Other

8. Do you believe your medical society/societies should be educating the public about the loss of the cerebral cortex, the seat of all human characteristics (the permanent vegetative state)?
   Yes   No

9. Do you believe it would be helpful to add to the criteria of death the absence of cerebral function?
   Yes   No

10. Do you believe that the physician community has a responsibility to our society to use health care resources wisely?
    Yes   No

    If yes: Is that happening now?
    Yes   No

11. Does this statement sound right to you?
    Autonomy means patients have the right to refuse appropriate care, no physician should offer and no patient/family can demand inappropriate care. Appropriate care is beneficial, supported by best available medical evidence taking into account patients overall health and age.
    Yes   No

12. Have you found that over the years consumerism and the possibility of legal action have caused you or your colleagues to provide nonbeneficial care?
    Yes   No

13. Would it help if your medical society had a local panel of physicians, nurses, clergy, and a public representative available for support in difficult situations (to help unify standards of care)?
    Yes   No

    What society/societies should be involved?
    — AMA
    — ACP
    — ACS
    — CANeurology
    — Other(s)

14. In your opinion, are healthcare costs in America pricing many of our goods out of the global market?
    Yes   No

    Do physicians have a responsibility in this area?
    Yes   No

15. Do you think hospital/health care administrations want physicians to use billable technologies?
    Yes   No

    If yes, do you think there are subtle messages encouraging the use of these technologies?
    Yes   No

16. In the course of your career are you now seeing more aggressive end-of-life care that is inhibiting referral to hospice?
    Yes   No

17. Please add any further comments or observations.

POLITICAL LEADERS SURVEY

1. Do you receive your medical care in the United States?
   Yes   No

2. Do you believe that our medical system delivers excellent end-of-life care?
   Yes   No

   If no, the reason(s) is/are (check all that apply):
   — Too frequent use of technology
   — Lack of humane care
   — Inappropriate use of hospital facilities
   — Protracted dying
   — Too expensive
   — Lack of physician skill
   — Controlling symptoms
   — Grief counseling with family
   — Acting as if afraid of lawsuits
   — Overuse of technology
   — Lack of concern for society's resources

3. Do you believe the public is satisfied with our nation's end-of-life care?
   Yes   No

   If no, the reason(s) is/are (check all that apply):
   — Too frequent use of technology
   — Lack of humane care
   — Inappropriate use of hospital facilities
   — Protracted dying
   — Too expensive
   — Lack of physician skill
   — Controlling symptoms
   — Grief counseling with family
   — Acting as if afraid of lawsuits
   — Overuse of technology
   — Lack of concern for society's resources

4. In your opinion, if there is a problem with end-of-life care in the United States, what are the reasons it is not being addressed?
   — Medicare is so vast and expensive nobody knows what and where to fix it.
   — Dying is a taboo subject; nobody wants to talk about it.
   — We in the United States love technology, and thus it is difficult to not use it.
   — Our medical system as presently constituted needs to use technology to sustain itself financially.
   — Physicians have, in many cases, lost the skill to use technology wisely.
   — There is an irrational fear of lawsuits.
   — We have relegated end-of-life care to nursing homes which are ill equipped to deal with this phase of life.
   — Many hospitals depend on nursing home patients to maintain cash flow regardless as to the wisdom of which patients to treat using Intensive Care Units, etc.
   — There is an inadequate use of hospice, hospice home care, or comfort care facilities vs. medically oriented nursing homes.
   — Other.

5. Should Congress adjust Medicare/Medicaid laws to discourage hospital end-of-life care and encourage hospice?
   Yes   No

6. Are our (U.S.) healthcare costs putting an additional burden on our manufacturing base, causing us to be at a disadvantage globally?
   Yes   No

   If yes, do you believe this is causing us to lose manufacturing jobs?
   Yes   No

7. Do you think it would be wise for the medical community to try to develop a definition of death that would include permanent loss of the cerebral cortex (the seat of the human spirit)? This would end the controversy around the permanent vegetative state.
   Yes   No

8. Do you think it would be helpful if medical societies had in place local committees with physicians, nurses, clergy, and lay representation to support physicians and hospital ethics committees to help resolve contentious end-of-life disputes (this would help coordinate standards of care)?
   Yes   No

   If yes, do you think Medicare should help fund this process?
   Yes   No

9. Administrative costs for American medicine are about 20 percent of total expenses versus 5 percent for other developed countries. Would you be in favor of creating a single consortium for billing and electronic medical records?
   Yes   No

10. Please feel free to make any further comments or suggestions about improving American medicine.

Appendix 2

Family-Physician Interactions

DISCUSSION POINTS PHYSICIANS SHOULD INITIATE IN END-OF-LIFE SITUATIONS

1. Identify those patients that may be nearing the end of their lives. They may be terminal cancer patients, frail elderly patients who have been in and out of the hospital, or they may be patients with a chronic illness such as congestive heart failure who are experiencing more and more serious problems. Patients like these have a right to know what lies down the road, and just knowing what to expect can relieve a lot of anxiety and fear.

2. Talk with them about their concerns. Perhaps it is fear of pain, or of being unable to care for themselves. Perhaps they are alone with no family support. You can begin the process of educating them about palliative care and hospice, and about community-based support programs.

3. Talk to them about unexpected events they have experienced in the course of their disease. Perhaps they had an episode of breathing difficulty that was unanticipated. You can make plans to meet future events, and reassure both patient and family in the process.

4. Bring up the subject of advance directives, and who can speak for patients if they can't speak for themselves. An advance directive should be completed in the later stages of the disease process, not years before, so that it is recent and timely. Advanced directives advise the medical community of what indicated procedures or technology the patient does not want, including their right to forgo palliative care, and accept whatever nature has to offer.

5. Since most of us would be more comfortable at home, educate the patient and the family about services and programs that are available.

6. Discuss treatments and procedures that will benefit the patient, and bring quality of life at the end, not just treatment for treatment's sake so that everyone can say "we did everything we could."

QUESTIONS FAMILIES SHOULD ASK IN END-OF-LIFE SITUATIONS

1. What are the chances the patient will leave the hospital alive and have an acceptable level of human function? Level of function may vary from

patient to patient. However, complete lack of human function means it might be time to make a tough decision. Human function may be defined as an ability to communicate in some way, possess some mobility that enables at least minimal independence, and have an acceptable degree of cognitive function that reflects awareness of the world and self. These are all cerebral functions.

2. What about some of the grading systems that have been developed? What is the patient's score and what does that mean for survival?

3. As days pass, what progress is being made? Is the patient declining, improving, or staying the same? What is the trend? This trend should become obvious over the course of a few days to a week.

4. Is this an acute problem that has a better chance of improvement, or is it a progressive chronic situation?

5. Is there permanent and complete loss of the cerebral cortex (blood flow scans)? (With no cerebral cortical function there is no human activity, such as thinking, purposeful movement, purposeful communication, etc.)

6. Does an acute care facility have anything positive to offer, considering the overall condition of this patient?

7. Is it time for palliative care and hospice? Should there be a consultation with the palliative care team to determine if this would be appropriate? Is the patient undergoing suffering that will have no benefit?

Appendix 3

The Baby K Case

ASKING THE COURTS TO SET THE STANDARD OF EMERGENCY CARE—THE CASE OF BABY K[*]

George J. Annas

Almost two decades ago, Dr. Franz J. Ingelfinger predicted that if physicians kept turning to the courts "to resolve essentially medical matters," the medical profession's unfortunate "dependence on the lawyer in reaching essentially medical decisions will continue."[1] One can argue about what decisions are "essentially medical," but the trend that worried Dr. Ingelfinger has continued, and now physicians and a hospital have sought legal and judicial guidance about how—and whether—to treat an anencephalic infant known as Baby K.

TREATING BABY K

Baby K was born by cesarean section on October 13, 1992, at Fairfax Hospital in Falls Church, Virginia. Anencephaly was diagnosed prenatally, and her mother decided to continue the pregnancy despite recommendations for termination from both the obstetrician and a neonatologist. The newborn had difficulty breathing at birth, and mechanical ventilation was begun. Within days the physicians began urging the mother (the father was only distantly involved) to agree to discontinue ventilation, since it served no therapeutic or palliative purpose and was therefore medically inappropriate. The mother refused. The physicians turned to the hospital's ethics committee and met with a subcommittee composed of a family practitioner, a psychiatrist, and a minister. On October 22 the subcommittee concluded that if the impasse between the physicians and the mother continued, a legal resolution should be sought.

Baby K was transferred to a nursing home on November 30, a time when she was not dependent on mechanical ventilation. Her mother agreed to the transfer on condition that the hospital would take the baby back if her respiratory

[*]*New England Journal of Medicine*, Vol. 330: 1542–1545, May 26, 1994, number 21.
Copyright © 1994 Massachusetts Medical Society. All rights reserved. Reprinted with permission.

difficulties recurred. On January 15, 1993, Baby K returned to the hospital for ventilatory support and stayed there until February 12. She has returned at least twice since. At this time she continues to reside at the nursing home. Assuming her diagnosis is correct, she may be the longest-lived anencephalic infant in medical history.[2]

Fairfax Hospital went to federal court seeking a ruling that it was not obligated to render "inappropriate" medical treatment to Baby K under existing federal and state law should Baby K again come to the emergency department in respiratory distress. The mother's position was that "all human life has value, including her anencephalic daughter's life."[3] She has "a firm Christian faith . . . [and] believes that God will work a miracle if that is his will. . . . God, and not other humans, should decide the moment of her daughter's death."[3] The hospital, the guardian ad litem appointed by the court, and Baby K's father all believed that further ventilatory assistance to Baby K was medically and ethically inappropriate.

THE OPINION OF THE TRIAL COURT

The trial judge, District Court Judge Claude Hilton, focused almost exclusively on antidiscrimination legislation in his opinion. Under the Examination and Treatment for Emergency Medical Condition and Women in Active Labor Act (Emergency Treatment Act), enacted by Congress to prevent the arbitrary refusal of treatment to uninsured people ("patient dumping"), all hospitals with emergency departments that receive Medicare funds must treat any person who arrives with an emergency medical condition and must continue treatment until the person's condition is stabilized and the person can be safely transferred.[4] Fairfax Hospital conceded that respiratory distress was an emergency condition but argued that the statute should be interpreted to include an exception for treatment deemed "futile" or "inhumane" by the hospital physicians. The judge disagreed for two reasons: first, the statute did not contain this exception, and second, even if it did, the exception would not apply to Baby K because her breathing could be restored; therefore, mechanical ventilation could not be considered either futile or inhumane. The judge added:

> To hold otherwise would allow hospitals to deny emergency treatment to numerous classes of patients, such as accident victims who have terminal cancer or AIDS, on the grounds that they eventually will die anyway from those diseases and that emergency care for them would therefore be "futile."[3]

Judge Hilton also ruled that section 504 of the Rehabilitation Act[5] and the Americans with Disabilities Act[6] both prohibited discrimination against Baby K based on her anencephaly. Finally, the judge ruled that as a general matter of law, "absent a finding of neglect or abuse," parents have the right to make decisions about medical treatment for their children.[3] When parents disagree with each other, the judge concluded that the courts should support the parent who decides "in favor of life."[3]

THE COURT OF APPEALS

On February 10, 1994, the U.S. Court of Appeals, in a two-to-one opinion, affirmed the July 1993 judgment of the trial court.[7] The appeals court, however, examined only one question in reaching its decision: Did Congress, in passing the Emergency Treatment Act, provide an exception for anencephalic infants (or anyone else) in respiratory distress? The court found the language of the statute clear and unambiguous: hospitals are required to stabilize the medical condition creating the emergency. In the court's words, "a straightforward application of the statute obligates the hospital to provide respiratory support to Baby K when she arrives at the emergency department of the hospital in respiratory distress and treatment is requested on her behalf."[7]

In making its case, the hospital suggested four reasons why the rule should not apply to Baby K, all of which were rejected. Two of the reasons merit discussion. The first was that Baby K's emergency condition was not respiratory distress, but anencephaly. The court disagreed, noting that it was her respiratory distress, not her anencephaly, that brought her to the emergency department. Second, the hospital argued that Congress did not "intend to require physicians to provide medical treatment outside the prevailing standard of medical care" in passing the Emergency Treatment Act. The appeals court seemed to agree with the hospital that the "prevailing standard of medical care for infants with anencephaly is to provide only warmth, nutrition, and hydration."[7] Nonetheless, the court held that the statutory language was "unambiguous" and included no such limitation on the hospital's responsibility to stabilize emergency conditions:

> We recognize the dilemma facing physicians who are requested to provide treatment they consider morally and ethically inappropriate, but we cannot ignore the plain language of the statute because "to do so would transcend our judicial function. . . . The appropriate branch to redress the policy concerns of the Hospital is Congress."[7]

Later in its decision the appeals court reiterated the point: "It is beyond the limits of the court's judicial function to address the moral or ethical propriety of providing emergency stabilizing medical treatment to anencephalic infants."[7] The court concluded that the Emergency Treatment Act makes no exception either for such infants or for

> comatose patients, those with lung cancer, or those with muscular dystrophy— all of whom may repeatedly seek emergency stabilizing treatment for respiratory distress and also possess an underlying medical condition that severely affects their quality of life and ultimately may result in their death.[7]

The dissenting judge argued that the Emergency Treatment Act was enacted to prevent patients from being dumped for economic reasons and that since dumping was not an issue with Baby K, the statute was irrelevant. He also argued that it was wrong to consider Baby K's treatment as involving a series of discrete emergency conditions; rather, her care should be "regarded as a continuum," since there is "no medical treatment that can improve her condition [of permanent unconsciousness]."[7]

MIXED MESSAGES AND CONFUSED ROLES

Many misjudgments were made in this case, but all relate to the failure to distinguish among medical standards, ethical precepts, and legal requirements. After birth Baby K was given mechanical ventilation. This was a medical misjudgment (assuming the physicians really believed it was medically inappropriate) that may have given the mother the impression that the doctors would provide medically inappropriate treatment to her child if she so desired. Since the physicians had known for months that she would be delivering an anencephalic baby, the issue of mechanical ventilation should have been resolved with the mother before the birth. If the physicians believed (on the basis of medical standards) that mechanical ventilation was contraindicated, the mother should have been informed that it would not be used and given an opportunity to find alternative care givers. If ventilation was to be used, the goal of this intervention (e.g., to confirm the diagnosis) should have been clearly specified, and support should have continued only until the goal was reached or was found to be unattainable.[8]

The ethics subcommittee at the hospital also misconstrued its role. It seems to have discussed nothing ethical at all. Composed of two physicians and a minister, it gave advice on medical practice and legal strategy, concluding that if the physicians could not reach agreement with the mother, the hospital should seek judicial relief. The subcommittee should have insisted that discussion with the mother continue until a resolution was reached, and it should have tried to facilitate this communication.

The hospital's administration and attorney seem also to have overreacted, though much more predictably. Instead of supporting their physicians in their application of existing medical standards or encouraging further discussion with the mother, they decided to go to court, because they saw Baby K's ventilatory support as a legal issue that might affect the institution, rather than an issue of medical practice or medical ethics.

The chief misjudgment by the trial judge was to try to act like a physician. His opinion can best be understood as that of a medical consultant who believes he has been asked one technical question: Can ventilatory support help an anencephalic infant in respiratory distress breathe more easily? His answer was yes.

The judge viewed this as a case of arbitrary discrimination by physicians against a mentally handicapped patient. He was correct that hospitals with emergency departments must provide medically appropriate treatment to stabilize the condition of all emergency patients. The physicians' desire not to give Baby K ventilatory support was, however, explained not by prejudice or financial concern, but instead by adherence to reasonable medical standards. Thus, the judge was chillingly wrong to equate Baby K (and anencephalic infants as a class) with patients with cancer or AIDS who are injured in automobile accidents. It is because of her anencephaly itself that Baby K cannot benefit from any medical intervention.[2] Patients with AIDS or cancer can, of course, benefit from emergency treatment.

To treat Baby K is not, however, inhumane (as the physicians argued), since she can neither feel pain nor suffer. But it is degrading to treat her for either our own symbolic purposes or those of her mother, because to do so is to treat her as an object—as a means to someone else's ends.[9] If the mere maintenance of biologic functioning in the absence of cortical function (vitalism) were a reasonable medical goal, physicians would be prohibited from ever discontinuing cardiopulmonary resuscitation in any patient, since it maintains circulation and ventilation. Nor has the judgment about treating anencephalic infants been made only by physicians. Congress and the executive branch have also been involved—the "Baby Doe regulations," for example, specifically recognized limits on care and the role of reasonable medical judgment in setting those limits.[9,10,11] The regulations themselves specified, and Surgeon General C. Everett Koop agreed, that a decision not to treat an anencephalic newborn is not discriminatory if based on a "legitimate medical judgment" that treatment would be "futile," because such treatment would "do no more than temporarily prolong the act of dying."[12,13] A parental request for treatment does not alter the physician's obligation to exercise reasonable medical judgment. The Child Abuse Amendments of 1984 are also consistent with this view.

By the time the case reached the more rarefied atmosphere of the Court of Appeals, the outcome was predictable. In answering its narrow question about the reach of the Emergency Treatment Act, the appeals court was correct: Congress provided no exceptions for anencephalic infants. On the other hand, I think the hospital was also correct in asserting that Congress did not intend to require physicians to provide emergency care "outside the prevailing standard of medical care." Certainly, neither side could point to any statute by which Congress has ever required physicians to violate existing standards of medical care. Nor is there any evidence that Congress intended to amend or in any way change the Baby Doe rules when it enacted the Emergency Treatment Act. It seems that the appeals court simply believed that the trial court had not acted unreasonably in favoring a mother who wanted her child treated over a hospital that wanted the child to die sooner rather than later.

THE ROLE OF MEDICAL STANDARDS

The logic of the Emergency Treatment Act as interpreted by these courts, although understandable in context, is incorrect because the technological imperative is limitless. To avoid cases like this one, Congress should have included the phrase "consistent with reasonable medical standards" in its requirement for stabilization. If the legal rule really were that hospitals and physicians had to provide any and all life-saving treatments to anencephalic infants that were wanted by the parents, they could be required to provide not only ventilatory support, but also other types of support, such as kidney dialysis for renal failure, and ultimately a heart-assist device when the child's heart begins deteriorating. As the dissenting judge properly argued, the focus must be on the patient as a person, not on the patient as reduced to a group of separate organ systems.

It is true that parents have (and should have) wide discretion in choosing among treatment options for their children. In the absence of evidence that a particular decision constitutes child abuse or neglect, we should presume that families can make the best decisions for their children. But it does not follow that physicians must do whatever parents (or adult patients themselves) order them to do regardless of standards of medical practice. Parents can choose among medically reasonable treatment alternatives, but they cannot prescribe treatment or demand that they or their children be mistreated.[14]

In the leading Supreme Court case cited by the trial judge, the Court upheld a state statute that permitted parents to commit a minor child to a mental institution without first providing the child with a court hearing.[15] But it did so only because the Court believed that the psychiatrist at the institution would act in the best interests of the child and not admit him or her unless the psychiatrist made an independent medical assessment that institutional care was in the child's best interests.[9,15] In another case, the Court ruled that retarded persons in state custody have a constitutional right to habilitation but that the content of that right should be left to the judgment of medical professionals.[16]

Thus, it is not the law that physicians must do whatever parents want. Rather, the law that parents should usually consent to treatment decisions made for their children is based on the premise that physicians will exercise independent medical judgment and not follow parental orders if the physician believes they are not in the best interest of the child or patient. In passing the Emergency Treatment Act, Congress was responding to situations in which physicians were refusing to treat patients in emergencies for economic reasons—not because of an exercise of medical judgment or standards of medical practice.

Because medicine has become a consumer good in many respects, and because many physicians and hospitals treat medicine as a business in which medical services are provided on the basis of the patient's desires rather than medical indications, it is becoming more and more difficult for physicians to refuse whatever patients and their families demand. Thus, for example, it is impossible for physicians to argue credibly that treating patients in persistent vegetative states is contrary to standards of medical practice, because most physicians actually provide continuing treatment if the family insists[17,18]. Treating medical care as a consumer good is a central reason why medical costs are out of control and why a national health plan that gives physicians financial incentives not to treat seems attractive to many policy makers.

WHAT SHOULD BE DONE?

Before the case of Baby K, the medical standard of practice was to provide no artificial ventilation to anencephalic infants. Now, physicians in emergency departments are legally obligated to provide assistance, ventilatory and otherwise, to anencephalic infants who need it to survive. Emergency physicians can live with this rule, because the case is not likely to arise again.

There are three possible scenarios for the future. In the first, physicians will do whatever patients want (as long as they can pay for it), because medicine will be seen as a consumer commodity like breakfast cereal and toothpaste. This will make medicine even more unbearably expensive than it is. Therefore, the second scenario, a variation on Dr. Ingelfinger's vision, is more likely. The task of defining "appropriate medical care" will be removed from physicians altogether and put in the hands of payers and government regulators, who will decide the content of medicine.

To avoid either of these scenarios, physicians must work toward a third, in which they not only set standards for medical practice, but also follow them. Physicians cannot expect parents, trial-court judges, insurance companies, or government regulators to take practice standards more seriously than they do themselves. If physicians cannot set standards for the treatment of anencephalic infants and adhere to them, standard-setting by physicians is a dead issue.

REFERENCES

1. Ingelfinger FJ. Legal hegemony in medicine. N Engl J Med 1975;293:825–826. [Medline]

2. The Medical Task Force on Anencephaly. The infant with anencephaly. N Engl J Med 1990;322:669–674. [Medline]

3. In the Matter of Baby K, 832 F.Supp. 1022 (E.D. Va. 1993).

4. Emergency Medical Treatment and Active Labor Act, P.L. 99-272, 42 U.S.C. sec. 1395dd (1985) (renamed in 1989).

5. Rehabilitation Act of 1973, P.L. 93-112, 29 U.S.C. sec. 701–796i (1973).

6. Americans with Disabilities Act, P.L. 101-336, 42 U.S.C. sec. 12101–12213 (1990).

7. In the Matter of Baby K, 16 F.3d 590 (4th Cir. 1994).

8. Paris JJ, Schreiber MD, Statter M, Arensman R, Siegler M. Beyond autonomy—physicians' refusal to use life-prolonging extracorporeal membrane oxygenation. N Engl J Med 1993;329:354–357. [Free Full Text]

9. Elias S, Annas GJ. Reproductive genetics and the law. Chicago: Year Book, 1987.

10. United States v. University Hospital, State University of New York at Stony Brook, 729 F.2d 144 (2d Cir. 1984).

11. Office of Human Development Services, Dept. Health & Human Services. Child abuse and neglect prevention and treatment program; final rule. Fed Regist 1985;50:14878–14901. [Medline]

12. Krushe H, Singer P. Should the baby live? New York: Oxford University Press, 1985.

13. Office of the Secretary, Department of Health and Human Services. Nondiscrimination on the basis of handicap relating to health care for handicapped infants; proposed rules. Fed Regist 1984;49:1621–1654.

14. Annas GJ. Judging medicine. Clifton, N.J.: Humana Press, 1988.

15. *Parham v. J.L. and J.R.*, 442 U.S. 584 (1979).

16. *Youngberg v. Romeo*, 457 U.S. 307 (1982).

17. Miles SH. Informed demand for "non-beneficial" medical treatment. N Engl J Med 1991;325:512–515. [Medline]

18. In re Wanglie, No. PX91-288 (Prob. Ct., Hennepin Co., Minn., June 28, 1991).

Appendix 4

In Support of Appropriate Care Committees

CARDIOLOGISTS GET WAKE-UP CALL ON STENTS[*]

Mike Mitka

Patients with stable coronary artery disease treated with stents and optimal medical therapy fare no better than those who receive optimal medical therapy alone, according to new findings from a large clinical trial. For many cardiologists, the results serve as a wake-up call that they need to reevaluate how frequently they offer stenting (which has slight risks associated with the intervention itself as well as stent-associated thrombotic events) as a first option for relief of stable angina. The data come from the Clinical Outcomes Utilizing Revascularization and Aggressive Drug Evaluation (COURAGE) trial, reported here in March at the annual conference of the American College of Cardiology.

* * *

"COURAGE brings us back to earth and gets rid of the irrational exuberance that surrounds stenting," said Steven Nissen, MD, immediate past president of the American College of Cardiology and medical director, Cleveland Clinic Cardiovascular Coordinating Center.

Today, more than 1 million stent procedures are performed in the United States and while estimates vary, up to 85% of these interventions are carried out on patients with stable coronary artery disease, the COURAGE investigators said.

Despite the considerable buzz surrounding the COURAGE trial, the investigators pointed out that the results confirm established guidelines issued by the American College of Cardiology and the American Heart Association, which state: ". . . there is no demonstrated survival advantage associated with revascularization in low-risk patients with chronic stable angina; thus, medical therapy should be attempted in most patients before considering percutaneous coronary intervention or coronary artery bypass grafting."

NOTES

1. Gibbons RJ et al. J AmColl Cardiol. 2003;41:159–168.A

GEOGRAPHICAL VARIATIONS IN MEDICARE SPENDING[*]

Editorial by Kenneth I. Shine, MD

Location, location, location. As in real estate, what you pay for health care varies significantly by where you make the purchase. But there is no guarantee that the quality of the product will vary with price.

In this issue, Fisher and colleagues[1,2] have provided compelling evidence that 5-year mortality rates, functional status, and quality of care for three conditions (acute myocardial infarction, hip fracture, and colorectal cancer) do not vary significantly from high-cost to low-cost hospital referral regions (HRRs). Costs varied primarily by the number of consultations, tests, and hospitalization days rather than by the evidence-based services required. If anything, mortality rates were somewhat greater in the highest-cost areas. There was wide variation in use of intensive care unit beds, emergency intubations, and feeding tubes during the last 3 years of life. Influenza and pneumococcal immunizations and Papanicolaou smears were performed less frequently in regions with higher expenditure indexes. Patients in areas with higher expenditure indexes were more likely to see medical subspecialists, and those in HRRs with lower expenditure indexes were more likely to see family practitioners. Although the differences are small, the authors point out some evidence that access to care was poorer in higher-expenditure areas.

This study is consistent with evidence that the more hospital beds, physicians, laboratories, and subspecialists are available in a region, the more they will be used.[3] Efforts in the United States to distribute physicians and beds more appropriately for the country's needs have met with limited success. However, our professional organizations must initiate efforts to help physicians and patients understand that more is not necessarily better. Where evidence is available for the proper approach to diagnosis and treatment, it should be applied appropriately. For conditions or circumstances in which evidence is not available, it must be collected. Evidence should drive diagnostic testing and treatment behaviors, and physicians must carefully examine the added value for the patient of each costly decision.

We know all too little about how clinical reasoning differs in regions with different health care expenditure patterns. Development of algorithms for treatment of a specific condition by physicians in high- and low-cost HRRs might be very revealing. Explicitly describing the decision tree (or clinical guidelines) would provide a mechanism for comparing how decisions vary from high- to low-expenditure areas. For example, do the indications for a procedure used in the care of a patient with myocardial infarction differ in different settings? The opportunity to observe the decision-making process for a number of standardized patients in various parts of the United States might characterize the process by which these remarkable variations come about.

The Institute of Medicine report *Crossing the Quality Chasm*[4] emphasized the need for "continuous healing relationships." A physician providing such a relationship has a responsibility to see that the patient receives appropriate evidence-based care but does not receive care that adds no value. The physician can advise on the number and nature of the subspecialists consulted and the frequency of examinations, tests, and procedures. The electronic medical record can have an important role in reducing redundant and unnecessary tests. The patient's continuing-care physician often is aware of which subspecialists practice cost-effectively. This information should influence referral recommendations. General internists and family physicians can integrate the care process and provide preventive services, which, as Fisher and colleagues show, are not as well provided in areas with large numbers of subspecialists. These physicians can play a crucial role in the appropriate use of intensive care unit beds and procedures at the end of life. These responsibilities emphasize further the importance of the involvement of a generalist physician in the care of every patient.

Clues in the work of Fisher and colleagues suggest that poorer access to care may increase costs. Patients in the most expensive HRRs had the lowest "global" satisfaction and the highest interpersonal satisfaction with care. This suggests that a patient who went to the doctor in the most expensive areas had a more meaningful interpersonal experience but that there was overall discomfort with a system that has large numbers of subspecialists, teaching hospitals, and so on. Reliance on emergency departments rather than on a continuing-care physician may delay the initiation of care. If, in fact, access is decreased in more expensive areas, it may lead to higher costs for care of patients coming later to care—and perhaps a slightly higher mortality rate. May delayed access result in increased services? This hypothesis deserves further exploration.

As Fisher and colleagues point out, if all 306 HRRs had the same costs as the lowest-cost HRRs, as much as 30% of health care costs might be eliminated without adversely affecting health care outcomes. We should test this hypothesis rather than assume that it is true. In the absence of professional leadership, and in the face of rising health care costs, insurers and policymakers could respond with increased co-payments for visits and nonpayment for tests and procedures that are not part of the evidence-based requirements. It would be far better for physicians to reduce the rate at which health care costs are increasing through more efficient care than to invite the blunt bludgeons of purchasers and insurers. Medical educators can work closely with students and house officers to define and redefine the need for visits, consultations, tests, and procedures. The challenge comes when these trainees see their own role models, who are largely subspecialists, maximizing the flow of patients and income. Do patients in such situations have a "continuous healing relationship"?

Fisher and colleagues have convincingly demonstrated that excellent outcomes for patients can be achieved in regions that do less, but do it right. The challenge is to convince the public that this is not about rationing but about better care. The last time the profession ignored rising health care costs, we got "managed care." Fisher and colleagues offer some clues that if carefully explored and elaborated might allow physicians to take a leadership role in controlling costs rather than wait for the next "market solution."

Kenneth I. Shine, MD RAND Arlington, VA 22202-5050
Dr. Shine is a cardiologist. He recently completed 10 years as the president of the Institute of Medicine of the National Academies. He now works on health security issues.

Requests for Single Reprints: Kenneth I. Shine, MD, RAND Corp., 1200 South Hayes Street, Arlington, VA 22202-5050. Ann Intern Med. 2003;138: 347–348.

REFERENCES

1. Fisher ES, Wennberg DE, Stukel TA, Gottlieb DJ, Lucas FL, Pinder EL. The implications of regional variations in Medicare spending. Part 1: The content, quality, and accessibility of care. Ann Intern Med. 2003;138:273–87.

2. Fisher ES, Wennberg DE, Stukel TA, Gottlieb DJ, Lucas FL, Pinder EL. The implications of regional variations in Medicare spending. Part 2: Health outcomes and satisfaction with care. Ann Intern Med. 2003;138:288–98.

3. Wennberg JE, Fisher ES, Skinner J. Geography and the debate over Medicare reform. Health Aff (Millwood). 13 February 2002. Available at www.healthaffairs.org/WebExclusives/Wennberg_Web_Excl_021302.htm.

4. Committee on Quality of Health Care in America. Crossing the Quality Chasm: A New Health System for the 21st Century. Washington, DC: Institute of Medicine–National Academy Pr; 2001.

PHYSICIAN-OWNED SPECIALTY HOSPITALS AND CORONARY REVASCULARIZATION UTILIZATION TOO MUCH OF A GOOD THING?[*]

Peter Cram, MD, MBA; Gary E. Rosenthal, MD

The emergence of specialty hospitals that focus on lucrative procedural aspects of medicine has generated a heated debate among policy makers[1,2] that largely

* Peter Cram, Gary E. Rosenthal, Physician-Owned Specialty Hospitals and Coronary Revascularization Utilization Too Much of a Good Thing? *Journal of the American Medical Association*, March 7, 2007; Vol. 297, no. 9. Copyright © 2007, American Medical Association. All rights reserved. Used with permission.

involves 4 issues: patient selection (i.e., "cherry-picking" of healthier and wealthier patients by specialty hospitals); quality of care in specialty and general hospitals; impact of specialty hospitals on the financial health of general hospitals; and influence of specialty hospitals on utilization and health care costs.

* * *

In this issue of JAMA, Nallamothu and colleagues[3] provide intriguing new data suggesting that increases in the use of coronary revascularization were 2.5 to 3 times higher in health care markets that experienced entry of a new physician-owned specialty hospital compared with markets without specialty hospitals, including those markets in which new revascularization programs were established at general hospitals. The differences reflected a much lower decline in use of coronary artery bypass graft surgery and a larger increase in use of percutaneous coronary intervention (PCI). The increase in PCI was particularly striking among patients without acute myocardial infarction, a group for whom PCI may provide less benefit, but that accounted for more than two thirds of all PCI procedures.

Alternatively, the growth in utilization in markets with new specialty hospitals may be directly attributable to procedures performed in the new specialty hospitals. Indeed, at the end of the observation period, in the study by Nallamothu et al, specialty hospitals had approximately twice the volume as new cardiac programs in general hospitals and accounted for more than a third of all revascularization procedures performed in their markets.

Even though it is not possible to dissect the fundamental drivers of utilization from the study by Nallamothu et al, or the influence of increased utilization on patient outcomes, the results need to be considered in light of 3 important issues currently confronting the US health care system. First, and perhaps most important, increasing evidence suggests a general lack of association between more aggressive management practices and greater health care expenditures and better patient outcomes at a population level.[4] At the individual patient level, the recently published Occluded Artery Trial (OAT) found that PCI performed more than 3 days following an acute myocardial infarction provided no benefits relative to medical therapy.[5] Yet payment policies promoted by Medicare and other third-party payers have created large financial incentives favoring procedural interventions over careful medical management and disease prevention.[6] These policies may change with the recently enacted update to the Medicare physician fee structure that will increase reimbursement for evaluation and management visits, while reducing reimbursement for many procedures, including PCI.[7,8] Changes in the relative reimbursement for cognitive and procedural services and further refining of prospective payment to more equitably reimburse hospitals that care for more complex patients would likely mitigate the financial incentives driving specialty hospital growth. Nonetheless, potential drivers of physician interest in specialty hospitals, other than financial motivation, must be recognized, including a desire by physicians to gain greater control over hospital operations and quality,[9] which, in turn, are related to the most fundamental issues of medical professionalism and physician job satisfaction.

Third, the results of the study by Nallamothu et al should be considered in light of the data on physician- and hospital- (or supply-) induced demand. Physician ownership of ancillary services has been associated with overuse of these services, raising questions about whether physicians are placing their own financial interests ahead of their patients' best interests.[10] This concern has provided the impetus for the federal ban on physician ownership of facilities such as pharmacies and home health agencies.[11] The current findings raise important questions about the appropriateness of the "whole hospital" exemption loophole that permits physician ownership of specialty hospitals.

Author Affiliations: Division of General Internal Medicine, Department of Internal Medicine, University of Iowa Carver College of Medicine, Iowa City, and Center for Research in the Implementation of Innovative Strategies for Practice (CRIISP), Iowa City Veterans Administration Medical Center, Iowa City, Iowa. Corresponding Author: Peter Cram, MD, MBA, Center for Research in the Implementation of Innovative Strategies in Practice, VA Iowa City Healthcare System, Highway 6 W, Iowa City, IA 52246-2208 (**peter-cram@uiowa.edu**).

REFERENCES

1. Wilson BC. My hospital was doomed. Wall Street Journal. January 5, 2006: 20.

2. Fong T. Not so special: doc ownership in specialty hospitals scrutinized by healthcare panel. Mod Healthc. 2003;33:20–21.

3. Nallamothu BK, Rogers MAM, Chernew ME, Krumholz HM, Eagle KA, Birkmeyer JD. Opening of specialty cardiac hospitals and use of coronary revascularization in Medicare beneficiaries. JAMA. 2007;297:962–968.

4. Nallamothu BK, Rogers MAM, Chernew ME, Krumholz HM, Eagle KA, Birkmeyer JD. Opening of specialty cardiac hospitals and use of coronary revascularization in Medicare beneficiaries. JAMA. 2007;297:962–968.

5. Hochman JS, Lamas GA, Buller CE, et al. Coronary intervention for persistent occlusion after myocardial infarction. N Engl J Med. 2006;355:2395–2407. 11. Leonhardt D. What's a pound of prevention really worth? New York Times. January 24, 2007:C1.

6. Leonhardt D. What's a pound of prevention really worth? New York Times. January 24, 2007:C1.

7. Center for Medicare & Medicaid Services. Medicare program; revisions to payment policies, five-year review of work relative value units. Fed Regist. 2006;71: 69623–70251.

8. Hayes KJ, Pettengill J, Stensland J. Getting the price right: Medicare payment rates for cardiovascular services. Health Aff (Millwood). 2007;26:124–136.

9. General Accounting Office. Report to the Congress: Physician-Owned Specialty Hospitals. Washington, DC: General Accounting Office; 2005:1–51.

10. Mitchell JM, Sass TR. Physician ownership of ancillary services: indirect demand inducement or quality assurance? J Health Econ. 1995;14:263–289.

11. O'Sullivan JO. Medicare: Physician self-referral ("Stark I and II"). 2004. http://www.law.umaryland.edu/marshall/crsreports/crsdocuments/RL32494.pdf. Accessed February 13, 2007.

HOW PHYSICIANS CAN CHANGE THE FUTURE OF HEALTH CARE*

Michael E. Porter, PhD, MBA;
Elizabeth Olmsted Teisberg, PhD, MEngr, MS

Today's preoccupation with cost shifting and cost reduction undermines physicians and patients. Instead, health care reform must focus on improving health and health care value for patients. We propose a strategy for reform that is market based but physician led. Physician leadership is essential. Improving the value of health care is something only medical teams can do.

The right kind of competition—competition to improve results—will drive dramatic improvement. With such positive-sum competition, patients will receive better care, physicians will be rewarded for excellence, and costs will be contained. Physicians can lead this change and return the practice of medicine to its appropriate focus: enabling health and effective care.

Three principles should guide this change:

1. The goal is value for patients,
2. Medical practice should be organized around medical conditions and care cycles, and
3. Results—risk-adjusted outcomes and costs—must be measured.

Following these principles, professional satisfaction will increase and current pressures on physicians will decrease. If physicians fail to lead these changes, they will inevitably face ever-increasing administrative control of medicine. Improving health and health care value for patients is the only real solution. Value-based competition on results provides a path for reform that recognizes the role of health professionals at the heart of the system.

Author Affiliations: Harvard University, Cambridge, Mass (Dr Porter); Darden Graduate School of Business, University of Virginia, Charlottesville (Dr Teisberg). Corresponding Author: Michael E. Porter, PhD, MBA, Institute for Strategy and Competitiveness, Harvard Business School, Soldiers Field Road, Boston, MA 02163 (**mporter@hbs.edu**).

FOR FURTHER READING

There are so many wonderful articles supporting the ideas presented in this book that it's sometimes tough to know where to start, and even tougher when to stop. The following list offers a short synopsis of articles or studies that you may find interesting, even shocking. I have provided full citations and directions for accessing them online.

Understanding the Moral Distress of Nurses Witnessing Medically Futile Care

This study was the result of a survey of nurses attending continuing education courses on end-of-life care. All participants expressed emotional distress in seeing futile treatment of dying patients, especially when the treatments caused greater suffering. Most felt that palliative care and patient comfort were overlooked in favor of needless and hopeless procedures.

Ferrell Betty R., RN. PhD, FAANI, Understanding the Moral Distress of Nurses Witnessing Medically Futile Care, *Oncology Nursing Forum*, Oncology Nursing Society, Volume 33, May 2006. Pages 922–930. PMID: 16955120. To access the full study, go to www.ncbi.nlm.nih.gov/entrez and type in the PMID number.

Use of Intensive Care at the End of Life in the United States: An Epidemiologic Study

This study found that 20% of end-of-life patients will die in an Intensive Care Unit. The authors conclude that in the coming years, the Baby Boomers will put incredible strain on services unless there is more stringent advanced care planning, and greater capability to care for dying patients in settings other than the hospital or ICU.

Angus DC, Barnato AE, Linde-Zwirble WT, Weissfeld LA, Watson RS, Rickert T, Rubenfeld GD; Robert Wood Johnson Foundation ICU End-Of-Life Peer Group. (Abstract) *Critical Care Medicine*, 2004. PMID: 15090940 [PubMed - indexed for MEDLINE] To access the full study, go to www.ncbi.nlm.nih.gov/entrez/querry/ and type in the PMID number.

Trends in Inpatient Treatment Intensity among Medicare Beneficiaries at the End of Life

This study found that even though there was a decrease in the numbers of Medicare beneficiaries dying in the hospital because more patients opted for hospice care, the cost of their care was still increasing. The authors found that of those patients that did die in the hospital, more of them received expensive procedures, more of them were admitted to Intensive Care Units more often, and CPR was performed more often.

Barnato AE, McClellan MB, Kagay CR, Garber AM. Trends in inpatient treatment intensity among Medicare beneficiaries at the end of life. (Abstract) *Health Service Research,* 2004. PMID: 15032959 [PubMed - indexed for MEDLINE]. To access the full study, go to http://www.ncbi.nlm.nih.gov/entrez/querry/ and type in the PMID number.

The Ethical Challenge and the Futile Treatment in the Older Population Admitted to the Intensive Care Unit

This study found that there was a higher rate of admission to Intensive Care Units in people over 60, with the highest admission rate for people between 70 and 79. They found that the older groups had longer stays in ICU, and death rates were higher. They conclude that physicians must be more diligent in determining if ICU admission is appropriate for end-of-life patients.

Frezza EE, Squillario DM, Smith TJ. (Abstract) *American Journal of Medical Quality* 1998;13:121–126. PMID: 9735474 [PubMed - indexed for MEDLINE]. To access the full study, go to http://www.ncbi.nlm.nih.gov/entrez/querry/ and type in the PMID number.

Changes in Critical Care Beds and Occupancy in the United States 1985–2000: Differences Attributable to Hospital Size

This study found that larger hospitals were increasing the number of critical care beds while reducing the number of regular care beds. This has serious implications for end-of-life patients who are often admitted to expensive critical care units when a more compassionate strategy would be palliative care in a less costly regular care bed.

Halpern NA, Pastores SM, Thaler HT, Greenstein RJ. Changes in critical care beds and occupancy in the United States 1985–2000: Differences attributable to hospital size. (abstract) *Critical Care Medicine*, 2006;34:2105–2112. PMID: 16755256 [PubMed - indexed for MEDLINE]. To access the full study, go to http://www.ncbi.nlm.nih.gov/entrez/querry/ and type in the PMID number.

Appendix 5

American Medical Education

AMERICAN MEDICAL EDUCATION 100 YEARS AFTER THE FLEXNER REPORT*

Molly Cooke, M.D., David M. Irby, Ph.D., William Sullivan, Ph.D., and Kenneth M. Ludmerer, M.D.

Medical education seems to be in a perpetual state of unrest. From the early 1900s to the present, more than a score of reports from foundations, educational bodies, and professional task forces have criticized medical education for emphasizing scientific knowledge over biologic understanding, clinical reasoning, practical skill, and the development of character, compassion, and integrity.[1-4] How did this situation arise, and what can be done about it? In this article, which introduces a new series on medical education in the *Journal,* we summarize the changes in medical education over the past century and describe the current challenges, using as a framework the key goals of professional education: to transmit knowledge, to impart skills, and to inculcate the values of the profession.

ABRAHAM FLEXNER AND AMERICAN MEDICAL EDUCATION

Almost a century ago, Abraham Flexner, a research scholar at the Carnegie Foundation for the Advancement of Teaching, undertook an assessment of medical education in North America, visiting all 155 medical schools then in operation in the United States and Canada. His 1910 report, addressed primarily to the public, helped change the face of American medical education.[5-7] The power of Flexner's report derived from his emphasis on the scientific basis of medical practice, the comprehensive nature of his survey, and the appeal of his message to the American public. Although reform in medical education was already under way, Flexner's report fueled change by criticizing the mediocre quality and profit motive of many schools and teachers, the inadequate curricula and facilities at a number of schools, and the nonscientific approach to preparation

New England Journal of Medicine 355:1339–1344. September 28, 2006. Copyright © 2006 Massachusetts Medical Society. All rights reserved. Used with permission.

for the profession, which contrasted with the university-based system of medical education in Germany.

At the core of Flexner's view was the notion that formal analytic reasoning, the kind of thinking integral to the natural sciences, should hold pride of place in the intellectual training of physicians. This idea was pioneered at Harvard University, the University of Michigan, and the University of Pennsylvania in the 1880s but was most fully expressed in the educational program at Johns Hopkins University, which Flexner regarded as the ideal for medical education.[8] In addition to a scientific foundation for medical education, Flexner envisioned a clinical phase of education in academically oriented hospitals, where thoughtful clinicians would pursue research stimulated by the questions that arose in the course of patient care and teach their students to do the same. To Flexner, research was not an end in its own right; it was important because it led to better patient care and teaching. Indeed, he subscribed to the motto, "Think much; publish little."[9]

TRANSFORMATION OF MEDICINE IN THE 20TH CENTURY

The academic environment has been transformed since Flexner's day. In academic hospitals, research quickly outstripped teaching in importance, and a "publish or perish" culture emerged in American universities and medical schools. Research productivity became the metric by which faculty accomplishment was judged; teaching, caring for patients, and addressing broader public health issues were viewed as less important activities. Thus, today's subordination of teaching to research, as well as the narrow gaze of American medical education on biologic matters, represents a long-standing tradition.[8]

In addition to the shift in the importance of research relative to teaching and patient care, a transformation in the process of research on human disease has contributed to our current state of affairs. For the first half of the 20th century, a distinctive feature of American medical education was the integration of investigation with teaching and patient care. Teaching, clinical care, and investigation each served the others' purposes, because most research was based on the direct examination of patients. Gifted clinical investigators tended to be equally gifted as clinicians and clinical teachers. After 1960, however, as medical research became increasingly molecular in orientation, patients were bypassed in most cutting-edge investigations, and immersion in the laboratory became necessary for the most prestigious scientific projects. Clinical teachers found it increasingly difficult to be first-tier researchers, and fewer and fewer investigators could bring the depth of clinical knowledge and experience to teaching that they once had.[10]

The increasing turbulence of the health care environment in the past 20 years has generated a second set of conditions inimical to medical education as Flexner imagined it. Clinical teachers have been under intensifying pressure to increase their clinical productivity—that is, to generate revenues by providing care for paying patients.[11-13] As a result, they have less time available for teaching, often to their immense frustration. In addition, the harsh, commercial atmosphere of the marketplace has permeated many academic medical centers. Students hear institutional leaders speaking more about "throughput," "capture of market share," "units of service," and the financial "bottom line" than about the prevention and relief of suffering. Students learn from this culture that health care as a business may threaten medicine as a calling.

Thus we arrive at our current predicament: medical students and residents are often taught clinical medicine either by faculty who spend very limited time seeing patients and honing their clinical skills (and who regard the practice of medicine as a secondary activity in their careers) or by teachers who have little familiarity with modern biomedical science (and who see few, if any, academic rewards in leaving their busy practices to teach). In either case, many clinical teachers no longer exemplify Flexner's model of the clinician-investigator.

LEARNING MEDICINE AS PROFESSIONAL EDUCATION

All forms of professional education share the goal of readying students for accomplished and responsible practice in service to others. Thus, professionals in training must master both abundant theory and large bodies of knowledge; the final test of their efforts, however, will be not what they know but what they do. The purpose of medical education is to transmit the knowledge, impart the skills, and inculcate the values of the profession in an appropriately balanced and integrated manner.[14,15] In the apprenticeship model of medical training that prevailed into the mid-19th century, student physicians encountered this knowledge and these skills and values as enacted by their teachers in the course of caring for patients. How are knowledge, skills, and professional values represented in contemporary medical education?

The way in which students encounter the knowledge base of medicine has been profoundly influenced, as Flexner intended, by the assimilation of medical education into the culture of the university. Theoretical, scientific knowledge formulated in context-free and value-neutral terms is seen as the primary basis for medical knowledge and reasoning. This knowledge is grounded in the basic sciences; the academy accommodates less comfortably the practical skills and distinct moral orientation required for successful practice in medicine. However, Flexner had not intended that such knowledge should be the sole or even the predominant basis for clinical decision making.[5] Within 15 years after issuing his report, Flexner had come to believe that the medical curriculum overweighted the scientific aspects of medicine to the exclusion of the social and humanistic aspects. He wrote in 1925, "Scientific medicine in America—young, vigorous and positivistic—is today sadly deficient in cultural and philosophic background."[16] He undoubtedly would be disappointed to see the extent to which this critique still holds true.

Responsibility for the care of patients is a powerful stimulus for learning,[17] and active learning requires that clinical skills, both cognitive and procedural, be attained through the supervised provision of patient care. As Flexner recognized, medical novices require the opportunity to practice skills under the guidance of experienced teaching physicians until they attain a high level of proficiency.

Increasing attention to the quality of care, patient safety, and documentation of care enhances medical practice[18] but threatens to relegate trainees to the role of passive observer. Given that every patient deserves the best possible care, we are challenged to provide appropriate opportunities for experiential learning and practice while meeting the service demands of teaching hospitals. The educational mission of teaching hospitals is further compromised by the absence of performance standards and assessment methods that can clearly establish that learners are ready to advance to the next level of independence and challenge.

The moral dimension of medical education requires that students and residents acquire a crucial set of professional values and qualities, at the heart of which is the willingness to put the needs of the patient first. A generation ago, the hours worked served as a simple proxy for dedication to patients; now, an appropriate concern for the wellbeing of trainees and the safety of their patients demands a new understanding of what it means to be dedicated to one's patients.[19] Professional values are continuously exemplified and enacted in the course of medical education through role modeling, setting expectations, telling stories and parables, and interacting with the health care environment, not just in courses on ethics and patient–doctor communication. However, the values of the profession are becoming increasingly difficult for learners to discern; the conclusions they draw, as they witness the struggle of underinsured working people to obtain health care, marked differences in the use of expensive technologies in different health care environments, and their physician-teachers in complicated relationships with companies that make health care products, should concern us.

Not only has the knowledge base for medical practice hypertrophied since Flexner's day, but the delivery of care has also become vastly more complicated, and the expectations of the public higher. However, it has been difficult to integrate the new skills, knowledge, and attitudes required for proficient practice into medical education at both the predoctoral and residency levels. Although many students and residents are interested in learning about interprofessional teamwork, population health, and health policy and the organization of health services, these topics tend to be poorly represented in medical school and residency curricula. It can be hard to teach messy real-world issues, but practitioners need to understand how these issues affect their patients and how to interact with, and ultimately improve, an exceedingly complex and fragmented system to provide good patient care.

PREPARING PHYSICIANS FOR THE 21ST CENTURY

What can be done to bring the knowledge, skills, and values that must be imparted by medical education into better balance and to prepare outstanding physicians for the 21st century? As the articles in this series will illustrate, the solutions are apparent for some problems, but medical schools and the institutions that sponsor residency programs need to develop the will to implement them. Other problems are more complex, and their solutions more uncertain.

With respect to medical knowledge, the gaps between what we know about how people learn and how medicine is currently taught can be corrected. Cognitive psychology has demonstrated that facts and concepts are best recalled and put into service when they are taught, practiced, and assessed in the context in which they will be used.[20] Several decades of research on clinical expertise have elucidated the thinking of physicians as they evaluate signs and symptoms, select and interpret diagnostic tests, and synthesize data to develop clinical assessments and care plans; these insights can be shared with learners as well as their teachers.[21]

The acquisition of skills for practice requires radical transformation. Although the dictum "see one, do one, teach one" may have characterized the way in which clinical skills were learned in the past, it is now clear that for training in skills to be effective, learners at all levels must have the opportunity to compare their performance with a standard and to practice until an acceptable level of proficiency is attained. An appreciation of the importance of practice and the honest admission that neophytes cannot perform high-stakes procedures at an acceptable level of proficiency demand that we develop approaches to skills training that do not put our patients at risk in service to education. The use of increasingly sophisticated simulations and virtual reality offers physicians at all levels the opportunity to refresh skills and learn new ones in a safe practice environment. Educational methods that allow the demonstration of mastery at one level, with respect to both technique and judgment, before progression to the next level teach an important lesson in professionalism as well.

The groundwork that has been laid by explicit instruction in professionalism, combined with effective role modeling and attention to the hidden curriculum of the practice environment, can support the development of a comprehensive and sophisticated understanding of professional education.[22] Sociologists have noted the importance of socialization and implicit learning in the development of professional attitudes and behaviors.[23]

It has long been observed that assessment drives learning. If we care whether medical students and residents become skillful practitioners and sensitive and compassionate healers, as well as knowledgeable technicians, our approaches to the evaluation of learners must reach beyond knowledge to rigorously assess procedural skills, judgment, and commitment to patients. Self-assessment, peer evaluations, portfolios of the learner's work, written assessments of clinical reasoning, standardized patient examinations, oral examinations, and sophisticated simulations are used increasingly to support the acquisition of appropriate professional values as well as knowledge, reasoning, and skills. Rigorous assessment has the potential to inspire learning, influence values, reinforce competence, and reassure the public.[24]

Much of what we know about effective interventions is not translated from research settings into everyday patient care. Increasing emphasis is being placed on evidence-based practice, systems approaches, and quality improvement. Advances in these areas require the ability to integrate scientific discoveries and context-specific experimentation for the continuous improvement of the processes of medical practice. New paradigms that connect these processes are emerging, and they have the potential to revolutionize both the way in which people learn and the environment in which learning takes place.[25]

FINDING THE WILL TO CHANGE

The need for a fundamental redesign of the content of medical training is clear. In some instances, the road that needs to be taken is also clear—for example, more emphasis should be placed on the social, economic, and political aspects of health care delivery. However, curricular reform is never simple or easy, and "turf battles" are inevitable. The challenge is not defining the appropriate content but rather incorporating it into the curriculum in a manner that emphasizes its importance relative to the traditional biomedical content and then finding and preparing faculty to teach this revised curriculum.[26–28]

Reform of the process of clinical education is even more challenging; however, both regulatory and voluntary efforts are under way.[29,30] Some schools are developing clerkships that no longer focus solely on departmental inpatient services but instead include interdisciplinary approaches to the teaching of inpatient and outpatient care.[31,32] Long-term preceptorships or apprenticeships are being reestablished to ensure adequate observation, supervision, and mentoring of trainees. Proposed reforms of residency education in both medicine and surgery include shortened core rotations and earlier specialty training.[33–35] But who will do the teaching? Early experiments to identify, celebrate, and support a cadre of outstanding clinician-teachers, side by side with the laboratory-scientists and physician-scientists who are academic medicine's first-class citizens, hold promise for developing the innovative programs and providing the attentive supervision, assessment, and mentoring that beginning physicians need.[36]

A final problem is the financing of medical education.[23,37–39] Good teaching, whether it is conducted in the classroom, clinic, or hospital, requires time. Innovative approaches to teaching, progressive skills instruction, multitiered assessment, and support of the development of professionalism all require teachers who have the time to observe, instruct, coach, and assess their students and who also have time for self-reflection and their own professional development. Although the educational mission is expensive, many medical schools already possess the funds to support teaching properly, if they choose to use the funds for this purpose.[40]

One hundred years ago, Flexner's critique of medical education converted an evolutionary change already under way in North American medical education into a revolution. Medicine and the sciences underpinning it have made equally transformative advances since Flexner's report, and once again, our approach to education is inadequate to meet the needs of medicine. Ossified curricular structures, a persistent focus on the factual minutiae of today's knowledge base, distracted and overcommitted teaching faculty, archaic assessment practices, and regulatory constraints abound. These challenges threaten the integrated acquisition of technical knowledge and contextual understanding, the appropriately supervised mastery of practical skills, and the internalization of essential values that together make for an informed, curious, compassionate, proficient, and moral physician.

No one would cheer more loudly for a change in medical education than Abraham Flexner. He recognized that medical education had to reconfigure itself in response to changing scientific, social, and economic circumstances in order to flourish from one generation to the next. The flexibility and freedom to change— indeed, the mandate to do so—were part of Flexner's essential message. He would undoubtedly support the fundamental restructuring of medical education needed today. Indeed, we suspect he would find it long overdue.

Supported by the Carnegie Foundation for the Advancement of Teaching and the Atlantic Philanthropies.
No potential conflict of interest relevant to this article was reported.
We are indebted to Lee Shulman, Ph.D., for his thoughtful contributions.

REFERENCES

1. Training tomorrow's doctors: the medical education mission of academic health centers. New York: The Commonwealth Fund, 2002.

2. The Blue Ridge Academic Health Group. Reforming medical education: urgent priority for academic health center in the new century. Atlanta: Robert W. Woodruff Health Sciences Center, 2003.

3. Committee on the Roles of Academic Health Centers in the 21st Century. Academic health centers: leading change in the 21st century. Washington, DC: Institute of Medicine, 2003.

4. Educating doctors to provide high quality medical care: a vision for medical education in the United States. Washington, DC: Association of American Medical Colleges, 2004.

5. Flexner A. Medical education in the United States and Canada: a report to the Carnegie Foundation for the Advancement of Teaching. New York: Carnegie Foundation for the Advancement of Teaching, 1910.

6. Lagemann E. Private power for the public good: a history of the Carnegie Foundation for the Advancement of Teaching. Middletown, CT: Wesleyan University Press, 1983.

7. Bonner T. Iconoclast: Abraham Flexner and a life in learning. Baltimore: Johns Hopkins University Press, 2002.

8. Ludmerer K. Learning to heal: the development of American medical education. New York: Basic Books, 1985.

9. Flexner A. I remember: the autobiography of Abraham Flexner. New York: Simon and Schuster, 1940.

10. Ludmerer K. The internal challenges to medical education. Trans Am Clin Climatol Assoc 2003;114:241–53.

11. Tarquinio GT, Dittus RS, Byrne DW, Kaiser A, Neilson EG. Effects of performance-based compensation and faculty track on the clinical activity, research portfolio, and teaching mission of a large academic department of medicine. Acad Med 2003;78:690–701.

12. Williams RG, Dunnington GL, Folse JR. The impact of a program for systematically recognizing and rewarding academic performance. Acad Med 2003;78:156–66.

13. Berger TJ, Ander DS, Terrell ML, Berle DC. The impact of the demand for clinical productivity on student teaching in academic emergency departments. Acad Emerg Med 2004;11:1364–7.

14. Sullivan W. Work and integrity: the crisis and promise of professionalism in America. 2nd ed. San Francisco: Jossey-Bass, 2005.

15. Collins A, Brown J, Newman S. Cognitive apprenticeship: teaching the crafts of reading, writing and mathematics. In: Resnick L, ed. Knowing, learning and instruction: essays in honor of Robert Glaser. Hillsdale, NJ: Lawrence Erlbaum Associates, 1989:453–94.

16. Flexner A. Medical education: a comparative study. New York: MacMillan, 1925.

17. Miller J, Bligh J, Stanley I, al Shehri A. Motivation and continuation of professional development. Br J Gen Pract 1998; 48:1429–32.

18. Turning research into practice: cases on adopting evidence-based innovations for everyday care. Qual Lett Healthc Lead 2004;16(9):2–3, 5–9, 1.

19. Van Eaton EG, Horvath KD, Pellegrini CA. Professionalism and the shift mentality: how to reconcile patient ownership with limited work hours. Arch Surg 2005; 140:230–5.

20. Bransford J, Brown A, Cocking R. How people learn: brain, mind, experience, and school. Washington, DC: National Academy Press, 1999.

21. Norman G. Research in clinical reasoning: past history and current trends. Med Educ 2005;39:418–27.

22. Cruess RL, Cruess SR. Teaching medicine as a profession in the service of healing. Acad Med 1997;72:941–52.

23. Sinclair S. Making doctors: an institutional apprenticeship. Oxford, England: Berg, 1997.

24. Epstein RM, Hundert EM. Defining and assessing professional competence. JAMA 2002;287:226–35.

25. Berwick D. Escape fire: designs for the future of health care. San Francisco: Jossey-Bass, 2004.

26. Mennin SP, Kalishman S. Issues and strategies for reform in medical education: lessons from eight medical schools. Acad Med 1998;73:Suppl:S1–S64.

27. Davis AK, Kahn NB, Wartmann SA, Wilson M, Kahn R. Lessons from the Interdisciplinary Generalist Curriculum Project. Acad Med 2001;76:Suppl:S1–S157.

28. Pascoe JM, Cox M, Lewin LO, Weiss MD, Pye KL. Report on undergraduate medical education for the 21st century (UME-21): a national medical education project. Fam Med 2004;36:Suppl:S2–S150.

29. Leach DC. A model for GME: shifting from process to outcomes—a progress report from the Accreditation Council for Graduate Medical Education. Med Educ 2004;38:12–4.

30. Whitcomb ME. Redesigning clinical education: a major challenge for academic health centers. Acad Med 2005;80:615–6.

31. Speer AJ, Stagnaro-Green A, Elnicki DM. Interdisciplinary clerkships: educational models of the future? Am J Med 1995;99:451–3.

32. Harden R, Crosby J, Davis MH, Howie PW, Struthers AD. Task-based learning: the answer to integration and problem-based learning in the clinical years. Med Educ 2000;34:391–7.

33. DaRosa DA, Bell RH Jr, Dunnington GL. Residency program models, implications, and evaluation: results of a think tank consortium on resident work hours. Surgery 2003;133:13–23.

34. Goldman L. Modernizing the paths to certification in internal medicine and its subspecialties. Am J Med 2004;117:133–6.

35. Pellegrini CA, Warshaw AL, Debas HT. Residency training in surgery in the 21st century: a new paradigm. Surgery 2004; 136:953–65.

36. Dewey CM, Friedland JA, Richards BF, Lamki N, Kirkland RT. The emergence of academies of educational excellence: a survey of U.S. medical schools. Acad Med 2005;80:358–65.

37. Knapp R. Financing graduate medical education and limiting resident work hours: a political assessment. Am J Surg 2002;184:187–95.

38. Knapp RM. Complexity and uncertainty in financing graduate medical education. Acad Med 2002;77:1076–83.

39. Reinhardt UE. Academic medicine's financial accountability and responsibility. JAMA 2000;284:1136–8.

40. Ludmerer KM. Learner-centered medical education. N Engl J Med 2004;351: 1163–4.

Appendix 6

Pharmaceutical Company Issues

SURVIVING SEPSIS—PRACTICE GUIDELINES, MARKETING CAMPAIGNS, AND ELI LILLY[*]

Eichacker PQ, Natanson C, Danner RL

Practice guidelines approved by expert panels are intended to standardize care in such a way as to improve health outcomes. In recent years, the developers of such standards have started grouping evidence-based interventions into "bundles," on the theory that inducing physicians to follow multiple recommendations written into a single protocol has a measurable effect on patients' outcomes. As a side effect, bundled performance measures are readymade for use in pay-for-performance initiatives, which can base reimbursement on compliance with all the components.

Unfortunately, the development of such clusters is vulnerable to manipulation for inappropriate—and possibly harmful—ends. Seeing in these bundles a potentially powerful vehicle for promoting their products, pharmaceutical and medical-device companies have begun to invest in influencing the adoption of guidelines that serve their own financial goals. A case in point is the development of guidelines for the treatment of sepsis, which was orchestrated as an extension of a pharmaceutical marketing campaign.[1,2] Although its advocates viewed this effort as an important approach to reducing sepsis-related mortality, the campaign appears to have usurped guideline development for commercial purposes, possibly compromising highly regarded, third-party arbiters of medical quality in the process. Such intrusion into an initiative to benefit public health is of particular concern in this instance, since the drug incorporated into the performance measures was endorsed on the basis of a single controversial phase 3 trial that was still being called into question by additional studies even as the committee did its work.

In 2001, the Food and Drug Administration (FDA) approved Eli Lilly's Xigris (recombinant human activated protein C, or rhAPC, also known as drotrecogin

*New England Journal of Medicine 355:1640–1642. October 19, 2006. Copyright © 2006 Massachusetts Medical Society. All rights reserved. Used with permission.

alfa [activated]) for the treatment of sepsis. This approval was based primarily on a single phase 3 randomized, controlled trial—the Recombinant Activated Human Protein C Worldwide Evaluation in Severe Sepsis (PROWESS) study, published the same year—which showed a significant overall survival benefit at 28 days. The FDA acknowledged that there was controversy surrounding this decision, and half the members of the agency's advisory panel, pointing to methodologic and other important problems with the PROWESS study, voted to require that a confirmatory trial be performed before approval was granted. In its approval statement, the FDA recommended using rhAPC in patients deemed, on the basis of an Acute Physiology and Chronic Health Evaluation II score of 25 or more, to have a particularly high risk of death; since this criterion had not been prospectively validated, the agency asked Lilly to perform additional testing in selected subgroups. In the face of such uncertainty, initial sales of rhAPC fell short of market expectations (see timeline).[3]

To improve sales of rhAPC, in 2002, Lilly hired Belsito and Company, a public relations firm, to develop and help implement a three-pronged marketing strategy.[1] First, the product's sales were to be supported by marketing initiatives targeted to physicians and the medical trade media.[1] Second, because rhAPC was relatively expensive, word would be spread that the drug was being rationed and physicians were being "systematically forced" to decide who would live and who would die.[1,3] As part of this effort, Lilly provided a group of physicians and bioethicists with a $1.8 million grant to form the Values, Ethics, and Rationing in Critical Care (VERICC) Task Force, purportedly to address ethical issues raised by rationing in the intensive care unit.[3] Finally, the Surviving Sepsis Campaign was established, in theory to raise awareness of severe sepsis and generate momentum toward the development of treatment guidelines.

The first phase of the Surviving Sepsis Campaign was introduced at an October 2002 meeting of the European Society of Intensive Care Medicine (ESICM).

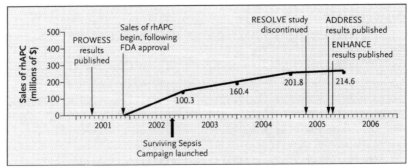

Timeline of Controlled Trials of rhAPC, Regulatory Actions, Yearly Sales, and the Marketing Initiative by Eli Lilly.

The Surviving Sepsis Campaign consisted of three phases — an initial one defining the need to treat sepsis, a second one developing treatment guidelines, and a third one developing and implementing performance bundles based on the guidelines. The four data points show end-of-year sales. The company had predicted annual sales of $300 million to $500 million.

In the second phase, launched in June 2003, international experts in critical care and infectious diseases were convened to create guidelines for sepsis management, which were published in *Critical Care Medicine* in March 2004.[4] Lilly provided more than 90% of the funding for these two phases, and many participants had financial or other relationships with the company.[1,4] According to the Council of Public Relations Firms, Belsito helped to assemble the VERICC Task Force and launch the campaign, and initiated a media-outreach program to "raise awareness" of alleged rationing in severe sepsis with the intent of generating demand for rhAPC.[1]

Campaign participants might argue that, regardless of Lilly's concerted efforts, the guidelines were not influenced by the company and represent best practice based on the evidence that was available—largely from randomized, controlled trials.[4] Although such trials represent the gold standard of medical evidence, overreliance on them in the construction of guidelines has a tendency to favor new drugs and devices, which typically undergo at least one such trial in order to obtain government approval. In this instance, that reliance meant that rhAPC was given a highly favorable rating (grade B), whereas established therapies for sepsis (such as antibiotics, fluids, and vasopressors), though included in the recommendations, received lower ratings (grade D or E), because most had not undergone randomized, controlled trials owing to a lack of equipoise.

This imbalance is made more troubling by the campaign's failure to discuss persisting concern about rhAPC, which has been reinforced by recent trials. After the PROWESS study, which had demonstrated an increased risk of serious bleeding, two other controlled trials—the Administration of Drotrecogin Alfa (Activated) in Early Stage Severe Sepsis (ADDRESS) study and the Resolution of Organ Failure in Pediatric Patients with Severe Sepsis (RESOLVE) study—both of which were terminated early because they were deemed unlikely to show a significant difference in their primary end points, confirmed that increase in risk and resulted in warnings submitted by Lilly to the FDA regarding the use of rhAPC. Although the results of the ADDRESS study were reported at the October 2004 ESICM meeting, no mention of the study was included in a supplement to the Surviving Sepsis Campaign Guidelines published the following month in *Critical Care Medicine*. Results from one open-label trial, the Extended Evaluation of Recombinant Human Activated Protein C (ENHANCE) study, published in October 2005, indicated that the risk of bleeding associated with rhAPC might actually be greater than originally estimated. Although data from the ENHANCE trial were available and are included in the guideline supplement, the possible magnitude of this increased risk (a 28-day incidence of serious bleeding of 6.5%, as compared with 3.5% in the PROWESS study) is not noted. Moreover, the efficacy of rhAPC has not been prospectively demonstrated in the patient population for which the drug is currently recommended.

Eleven professional societies are cited as sponsors of the Surviving Sepsis Campaign Guidelines. The Infectious Diseases Society of America (IDSA), however, declined to endorse them. According to Naomi O'Grady, the physician who chaired the IDSA's Standards and Practice Guidelines Committee from 2002 to

2005, the organization found fault with the manner in which the guidelines were developed, the use of a suboptimal rating system, and their sponsorship by a drug company. The peer-review process conducted by the IDSA might provide a model for an objective system of rating proposed guidelines in the future. But in this case, even the fact that the society decided not to endorse the recommendations is not widely known. According to Dante L. Landucci, an intensivist at East Carolina University, *Critical Care Medicine*, which published the guidelines, removed mention of the IDSA's rejection from his invited editorial on the subject that appeared in print 3 months after the guidelines did.

As part of the third phase of the campaign, Lilly awarded unrestricted grants for an "Implementing the Surviving Sepsis Campaign" program.[5] The main goal of this phase, launched in mid-2004, is the creation of performance bundles based on selected recommendations from the campaign guidelines. Again, many participants have self-reported financial or other relationships with Lilly.[4,5] Despite the persisting scientific controversy surrounding its safety and efficacy, rhAPC is included in one of these performance bundles. Neither the campaign's manual on bundle implementation nor a cover letter from the president of the Society of Critical Care Medicine mentions the ADDRESS and RESOLVE trials or the warnings they precipitated.[5] In formulating and promoting the bundles, the campaign sought to collaborate with public, not-for-profit arbiters of the quality of health care, including the Voluntary Hospital Association, the Institute for Healthcare Improvement, and the Joint Commission on Accreditation of Healthcare Organizations.[2,5]

Implementation of the bundles is being advocated nationally in workshops organized under the auspices of the Society of Critical Care Medicine and funded by Lilly. Furthermore, the campaign has lobbied state governments to adopt the bundles. Efforts to institute these measures internationally are being promoted in a program called the "Surviving Sepsis Campaign Roadshow," also subsidized by Lilly. In addition, the company funds *Advances in Sepsis*, a widely distributed periodical that publicizes the campaign. These activities continue unabated amid increasing calls for a new, prospective study of rhAPC.

When properly formulated and applied, practice guidelines and performance standards hold the promise of improving patients' outcomes. Professional societies and other stakeholders must work together to promote a consistent guideline-development process, a robust rating system for guidelines that is applicable to all subspecialties, and a policy that prohibits the pharmaceutical and medical-device industries from directly or indirectly funding or influencing practice standards. The challenges involved in producing firstrate guidelines and performance standards are only exacerbated by the intrusion of marketing strategies masquerading as evidence-based medicine.

Drs. Eichacker, Natanson, and Danner are senior investigators in the Critical Care Medicine Department, Clinical Center, National Institutes of Health, Bethesda, MD. The opinions expressed are those of the authors and do not reflect the policies of the National Institutes of Health, the Public Health Service, or the Department of Health and Human Services.

REFERENCES

1. Eli Lilly, Belsito. Surviving Sepsis: case studies—marketing communications of public relations firms. (Accessed September 28, 2006, at http://www.prfirms.org/resources/case_studies/Marketing_Communications/2004/SurvivingSepsis1.asp.)

2. Levy MM, Pronovost PJ, Dellinger RP, et al. Sepsis change bundles: converting guidelines into meaningful change in behavior and clinical outcome. Crit Care Med 2004;32: Suppl:S595-S597.

3. Regalado R. To sell pricey drug, Eli Lilly fuels a debate over rationing. Wall Street Journal. September 18, 2003:A1.

4. Dellinger RP, Carlet JM, Masur H, et al. Surviving Sepsis Campaign guidelines for management of severe sepsis and septic shock. Crit Care Med 2004;32:858-73. [Errata, Crit Care Med 2004;32:1448, 2169-70.]

5 National Institutes of Health. Online annotated bibliography for Surviving Sepsis—Practice Guidelines, Marketing Campaigns, and Eli Lilly. (Accessed September 28, 2006, at http://www.cc.nih.gov/ccmd/htmlpg/ccmsupplemental.html.)

Appendix 7

The Economic Impact of Our Healthcare If We Do Not Change

LONG-TERM CARE: AGING BABY BOOM GENERATION WILL INCREASE DEMAND AND BURDEN ON FEDERAL AND STATE BUDGETS*

Statement of David M. Walker, Comptroller General of the United States Before the Special Committee on Aging, U.S. Senate.

I am pleased to be here today as you discuss the effects of the aging baby boom generation on the demand for long-term care services and the challenges that increased demand will bring for federal and state budgets. In general, the aging of the baby boom generation will lead to a sharp growth in federal entitlement spending that, absent meaningful reforms, will represent an unsustainable burden on future generations. As the estimated 76 million baby boomers born between 1946 and 1964 become elderly, Medicare, Medicaid, and Social Security will nearly double as a share of the economy by 2035. We have been able to sustain these entitlements in the past with low depression-era birth rates and a large postwar workforce. However, absent substantive reform of entitlement programs, a rapid escalation of federal spending for Social Security, Medicare, and Medicaid beginning in less than 10 years from now is virtually certain to overwhelm the rest of the federal budget.

Most attention has been focused on the need for Social Security and Medicare reform in order to maintain their viability and ability to meet programmatic commitments. As I have testified before various committees, Social Security and Medicare's Hospital Insurance trust funds will face cash deficits not long after the first baby boomers are eligible to retire. While these are important issues, a broader focus should also include Medicaid, particularly as it involves financing long-term care. Long-term care includes an array of health, personal care, and supportive

*LONG-TERM CARE: *Aging Baby Boom Generation Will Increase Demand and Burden on Federal and State Budgets*, Statement of David M. Walker, Comptroller General of the United States Before the Special Committee on Aging, U.S. Senate, United States General Accounting Office Report, March 21, 2002.

services provided to persons with physical or mental disabilities. It relies heavily on financing by public payers, especially Medicaid, and has significant implications for state budgets as well as the federal budget.

My remarks today will focus on (1) the pressure that entitlement spending for Medicare, Medicaid, and Social Security is expected to exert on the federal budget in coming decades; (2) how the aging of the baby boom population will increase the demand for long-term care services; and (3) how these trends will affect the current and future financing of long-term care services, particularly in federal and state budgets. I will also highlight several considerations for any possible reforms of long-term care financing.

In summary, as more and more of the baby boom generation enters retirement over the coming decades, entitlement spending for Medicare, Medicaid, and Social Security is expected to absorb correspondingly larger shares of federal revenue and threatens to crowd out other spending. The aging of the baby boomers will also increase the demand for long-term care and contribute further to federal and state budget burdens. Estimates suggest the future number of disabled elderly who cannot perform basic activities of daily living without assistance may be double today's level. Current problems with the provision and financing of long-term care could be exacerbated by the swelling numbers of the baby-boom generation needing care. These problems include whether individuals with disabilities receive adequate services, the potential for families to face financially catastrophic long-term care costs, and the burdens and social costs that heavy reliance on unpaid care from family members and other informal caregivers create coupled with possibly fewer caregivers available in coming generations. Long-term care spending from all public and private sources, which was about $137 billion for persons of all ages in 2000, will increase dramatically in the coming decades as the baby boom generation ages. Spending on long-term care services just for the elderly is projected to increase at least two-and-a-half times and could nearly quadruple in constant dollars to $379 billion by 2050, according to some estimates. Without fundamental financing changes, Medicaid—which pays over onethird of long-term care expenditures for the elderly—can be expected to remain one of the largest funding sources, straining both federal and state governments.

In considering any long-term care financing reforms in light of these anticipated demands for assistance and budgeting stresses, it is important to keep in mind that long-term care is not just about health care. It also comprises a variety of services an aged and/or disabled person requires to maintain quality of life— including housing, transportation, nutrition, and social support to help maintain independent living. Given the challenges in providing and paying for these myriad and growing needs, several considerations for shaping reform proposals include:

- determining societal responsibilities;
- considering the potential role of social insurance in financing;
- encouraging personal preparedness;
- recognizing the benefits, burdens, and costs of informal caregiving;

- assessing the balance of state and federal responsibilities to ensure adequate and equitable satisfaction of needs;
- adopting effective and efficient implementation and administration of reforms; and
- developing financially sustainable public commitments.

BACKGROUND

Long-term care includes many types of services needed when a person has a physical or mental disability. Individuals needing long-term care have varying degrees of difficulty in performing some activities of daily living without assistance, such as bathing, dressing, toileting, eating, and moving from one location to another. They may also have trouble with instrumental activities of daily living, which include such tasks as preparing food, housekeeping, and handling finances. They may have a mental impairment, such as Alzheimer's disease, that necessitates supervision to avoid harming themselves or others or assistance with tasks such as taking medications. Although a chronic physical or mental disability may occur at any age, the older an individual becomes, the more likely a disability will develop or worsen.

According to the 1999 National Long-Term Care Survey, approximately 7 million elderly had some sort of disability in 1999, including about 1 million needing assistance with at least five activities of daily living. Assistance takes place in many forms and settings, including institutional care in nursing homes or assisted living facilities, home care services, and unpaid care from family members or other informal caregivers. In 1994, approximately 64 percent of all elderly with a disability relied exclusively on unpaid care from family or other informal caregivers; even among elderly with difficulty with five activities of daily living, about 41 percent relied entirely on unpaid care.

Nationally, spending from all public and private sources for long-term care for all ages totaled about $137 billion in 2000, accounting for nearly 12 percent of all health care expenditures.[1] Over 60 percent of expenditures for long-term care services are paid for by public programs, primarily Medicaid and Medicare. Individuals finance almost one-fourth of these expenditures out-of-pocket and, less often, private insurers pay for longterm care. Moreover, these expenditures do not include the extensive reliance on unpaid long-term care provided by family members and other informal caregivers.

Medicaid, the joint federal-state health-financing program for low-income individuals, continues to be the largest funding source for long-term care. Medicaid provides coverage for poor persons and to many individuals who have become nearly impoverished by "spending down" their assets to cover the high costs of their long-term care. For example, many elderly persons become eligible for Medicaid as a result of depleting their assets to pay for nursing home care that Medicare does not cover. In 2000, Medicaid paid 45 percent (about $62 billion) of total long-term care expenditures. States share responsibility with the federal government for Medicaid, paying on average approximately 43 percent of total Medicaid costs. Eligibility for Medicaid-covered long-term care services varies widely among states. Spending also varies across states—for example, in fiscal year 2000, Medicaid per capita long-term care expenditures ranged from $73 per year in Nevada to $680 per year in New York. For the national average in recent years, about 53 to 60 percent of Medicaid long-term care spending has gone toward the elderly. In 2000, nursing home expenditures dominated Medicaid long-term care expenditures, accounting for 57 percent of its long-term care spending. Home care expenditures make up a growing share of Medicaid long-term care spending as many states use the flexibility available within the Medicaid program to provide long-term care services in home- and community based settings.[2]

Expenditures for Medicaid home- and community-based services grew tenfold from 1990 to 2000—from $1.2 billion to $12.0 billion.

Other significant long-term care financing sources include:

- Individuals' out-of-pocket payments, the second largest payer of long-term care services, accounted for 23 percent (about $31 billion) of total expenditures in 2000. The vast majority (80 percent) of these payments were used for nursing home care.
- Medicare spending accounted for 14 percent (about $19 billion) of total long-term care expenditures in 2000. While Medicare primarily covers acute care, it also pays for limited stays in post-acute skilled nursing care facilities and home health care.
- Private insurance, which includes both traditional health insurance and long-term care insurance,[3] accounted for 11 percent (about $15 billion) of long-term care expenditures in 2000. Less than 10 percent of the elderly and an even lower percentage of the near elderly (those aged 55 to 64) have purchased long-term care insurance, although the number of individuals purchasing long-term care insurance increased during the 1990s.

ABSENT REFORM, SPENDING FOR MEDICAID, MEDICARE, AND SOCIAL SECURITY WILL PUT UNSUSTAINABLE PRESSURE ON THE FEDERAL BUDGET

Before focusing on the increased burden that long-term care will place on federal and state budgets, it is important to look at the broader budgetary context. As we look ahead we face an unprecedented demographic challenge with the aging of the baby boom generation. As the share of the population 65 and over climbs, federal spending on the elderly will absorb a larger and ultimately unsustainable share of the federal budget and economic resources. Federal spending for Medicare, Medicaid, and Social Security are expected to surge—nearly doubling by 2035—as people live longer and spend more time in retirement. In addition, advances in medical technology are likely to keep pushing up the cost of health care. Moreover, the baby boomers will be followed by relatively fewer workers to support them in retirement, prompting a relatively smaller employment base from which to finance these higher costs. Under the 2001 Medicare trustees' intermediate estimates, Medicare will double as a share of gross domestic product (GDP) between 2000 and 2035 (from 2.2 percent to 5.0 percent) and reach 8.5 percent of GDP in 2075. The federal share of Medicaid as a percent of GDP will grow from today's 1.3 percent to 3.2 percent in 2035 and reach 6.0 percent in 2075. Under the Social Security trustees' intermediate estimates, Social Security spending will grow as a share of GDP from 4.2 percent to 6.6 percent between 2000 and 2035, reaching 6.7 percent in 2075. Combined, in 2075 a full one-fifth of GDP will be devoted to federal spending for these three programs alone.

To move into the future with no changes in federal health and retirement programs is to envision a very different role for the federal government. Our long-term budget simulations serve to illustrate the increasing constraints on federal budgetary flexibility that will be driven by entitlement spending growth. Assume, for example, that last year's tax reductions are made permanent, revenue remains constant thereafter as a share of GDP, and discretionary spending keeps pace with the economy. Under these conditions, spending for net interest, Social Security, Medicare, and Medicaid would consume nearly three-quarters of federal revenue by 2030. This will leave little room for other federal priorities, including defense and education. By 2050, total federal revenue would be insufficient to fund entitlement spending and interest payments.[4]

Beginning about 2010, the share of the population that is age 65 or older will begin to climb, with profound implications for our society, our economy, and the financial condition of these entitlement programs. In particular, both Social Security and the Hospital Insurance portion of Medicare are largely financed as pay-as-you-go systems in which current workers' payroll taxes pay current retirees' benefits. Therefore, these programs are directly affected by the relative size of populations of covered workers and beneficiaries. Historically, this relationship has been favorable. In the near future, however, the overall worker-to-retiree ratio will change in ways that threaten the financial solvency and sustainability of these entitlement programs. In 2000, there were 4.9 working-age persons (18 to 64 years) per elderly person, but by 2030, this ratio is projected to decline to 2.8.[5] This decline in the overall worker-to-retiree ratio will be due to both the surge in retirees brought about by the aging baby boom generation as well as falling fertility rates, which translate into relatively fewer workers in the near future.

Social Security's projected cost increases are due predominantly to the burgeoning retiree population. Even with the increase in the Social Security eligibility age to 67, these entitlement costs are anticipated to increase dramatically in the coming decades as a larger share of the population becomes eligible for Social Security, and if, as expected, average longevity increases.

As the baby boom generation retires and the Medicare-eligible population swells, the imbalance between outlays and revenues will increase dramatically. Medicare growth rates reflect not only a rapidly increasing beneficiary population, but also the escalation of health care costs at rates well exceeding general rates of inflation. While advances in science and technology have greatly expanded the capabilities of medical science, disproportionate increases in the use of health services have been fueled by the lack of effective means to channel patients into consuming, and providers into offering, only appropriate services. Although Medicare cost growth had slowed in recent years, in fiscal year 2001 Medicare spending grew by 10.3 percent and is up 7.8 percent for the first 5 months of fiscal year 2002.

To obtain a more complete picture of the future health care entitlement burden, especially as it relates to long-term care, we must also acknowledge and discuss the important role of Medicaid. Approximately 71 percent of all Medicaid dollars are dedicated to services for the aged, blind, and disabled individuals, and Medicaid spending is one of the largest components of most states' budgets. At the February 2002 National Governors Association meeting, governors reported that during a time of fiscal crisis for states, the growth in Medicaid is creating a situation in which states are faced with either making major cuts in programs or being forced to raise taxes significantly. Further, in a 2001 survey, 24 states cited increased costs for nursing homes and home- and community-based services as among the top factors in Medicaid cost growth.[6] Over the longer term, the increase in the number of elderly will add considerably to the strain on federal and state budgets as governments struggle to finance increased Medicaid spending. In addition, this strain on state Medicaid budgets may be exacerbated by fluctuations in the business cycle, such as the recent economic slowdown. State revenues decline during economic downturns, while the needs of the disabled for assistance remain constant.

BABY BOOM GENERATION WILL GREATLY EXPAND DEMAND FOR LONG-TERM CARE

In coming decades, the sheer number of aging baby boomers will swell the number of elderly with disabilities and the need for services. These overwhelming numbers offset the slight reductions in the prevalence of disability among the elderly reported in recent years. In 2000, individuals aged 65 or older numbered 34.8 million people—12.7 percent of our nation's total population. By 2020, that percentage will increase by nearly one-third to 16.5 percent—one in six Americans—and will represent nearly 20 million more elderly than there are today. By 2040, the number of elderly aged 85 years and older—the age group most likely to need longterm care services—is projected to more than triple from about 4 million to about 14 million.

It is difficult to precisely predict the future increase in the number of the elderly with disabilities, given the counterbalancing trends of an increase in the total number of elderly and a possible continued decrease in the prevalence of disability. For the past two decades, the number of elderly with disabilities has remained fairly constant while the percentage of those with disabilities has fallen between 1 and 2 percent a year. Possible factors contributing to this decreased prevalence of disability include improved health care, improved socioeconomic status, and better health behaviors. The positive benefits of the decreased prevalence of disability, however, will be overwhelmed by the sheer numbers of aged baby boomers. The total number of disabled elderly is projected to increase to between onethird and twice current levels, or as high as 12.1 million by 2040.

The increased number of disabled elderly will exacerbate current problems in the provision and financing of long-term care services. Approximately one in five adults with long-term care needs and living in the community reports an inability to receive needed care, such as assistance in toileting or eating, often with adverse consequences.[7] In addition, disabled elderly may lack family support or the financial means to purchase medical services. Long-term care costs can be financially catastrophic for families. Services, such as nursing home care, are very expensive; while costs can vary widely, a year in a nursing home typically costs $50,000 or more, and in some locations can be considerably more. Because of financial constraints, many elderly rely heavily on unpaid caregivers, usually family members and friends; overall, the majority of care received in the community is unpaid. However, in coming decades, fewer elderly may have the option of unpaid care because a smaller proportion may have a spouse, adult child, or sibling to provide it. By 2020, the number of elderly who will be living alone with no living children or siblings is estimated to reach 1.2 million, almost twice the number without family support in 1990.[8] In addition, geographic dispersion of families may further reduce the number of unpaid caregivers available to elderly baby boomers.

SPENDING FOR LONG-TERM CARE FOR ELDERLY COULD NEARLY QUADRUPLE BY 2050

Currently, public and private spending on long-term care is about $137 billion for persons of all ages, and for the elderly alone is projected to increase two-and-a-half to four times in the next 40 to 50 years—reaching as much as $379 billion in constant dollars for the elderly alone, according to one source.[9] Estimates of future spending are imprecise, however, due to the uncertain effect of several important factors, including how many elderly will need assistance, the types of care they will use, and the availability of public and private sources of payment for care. Absent significant changes in the availability of public and private payment sources, however, future spending is expected to continue to rely heavily on public payers, particularly Medicaid, which estimates indicate pays about 36 to 37 percent of long-term care expenditures for the elderly.

One factor that will affect spending is how many elderly will need assistance. As I have previously discussed, even with continued decreases in the prevalence of disability, aging baby boomers are expected to have a disproportionate effect on the demand for long-term care. Another factor influencing projected long-term care spending is the type of care that the baby boom generation will use. Currently, expenditures for nursing home care greatly exceed those for care provided in other settings. Average expenditures per elderly person in a nursing home can be about four times greater than average expenditures for those receiving paid care at home.[10] The past decade has seen increases in paid home care as well as in assisted living facilities, a relatively newer and developing type of housing in which an estimated 400,000 elderly with disabilities resided in 1999.[11] It is unclear what effect continued growth in paid home care, assisted living facilities, or other care alternatives may have on future expenditures. Any increase in the availability of home care may reduce the average cost per disabled person, but the effect could be offset if there is an increase in the use of paid home care by persons currently not receiving these services.

Changes in the availability of public and private sources to pay for care will also affect expenditures. Private long-term care insurance has been viewed as a possible means of reducing catastrophic financial risk for the elderly needing long-term care and relieving some of the financial burden currently falling on public long-term care programs. Increases in private insurance may lower public expenditures but raise spending overall because insurance increases individuals' financial resources when they become disabled and allows the purchase of additional services. The number of policies in force remains relatively small despite improvements in policy offerings and the tax deductibility of premiums. However, as we have previously testified, questions about the affordability of long-term care policies and the value of the coverage relative to the premiums charged have posed barriers to more widespread purchase of these policies.[12]

Further, many baby boomers continue to assume they will never need such coverage or mistakenly believe that Medicare or their own private health insurance will provide comprehensive coverage for the services they need. If private long-term care insurance is expected to play a larger role in financing future generations' long-term care needs, consumers need to be better informed about the costs of long-term care, the likelihood that they may need these services, and the limits of coverage through public programs and private health insurance.

With or without increases in the availability of private insurance, Medicaid and Medicare are expected to continue to pay for the majority of long-term care services for the elderly in the future. Without fundamental financing changes, Medicaid can be expected to remain one of the largest funding sources for long-term care services for aging baby boomers, with Medicaid expenditures for long-term care for the elderly reaching as high as $132 billion by 2050. As I noted previously, this increasing burden will strain both federal and state governments.

CONSIDERATIONS FOR REFORMING LONG-TERM CARE FINANCING

Given the anticipated increase in demand for long-term care services resulting from the aging of the baby boom generation, the concerns about the availability of services, and the expected further stress on federal and state budgets and individuals' financial resources, some policymakers and advocates have called for long-term care financing reforms. As further deliberation is given to any long-term care financing reforms, I would like to close by suggesting several considerations for policymakers to keep in mind.

At the outset, it is important to recognize that long-term care services are not just another set of traditional health care services. Meeting acute and chronic health care needs is an important element of caring for aging and disabled individuals. Long-term care, however, encompasses services related to maintaining quality of life, preserving individual dignity, and satisfying preferences in lifestyle for someone with a disability severe enough to require the assistance of others in everyday activities. Some long-term care services are akin to other health care services, such as personal assistance with activities of daily living or monitoring or supervision to cope with the effect of dementia. Other aspects of long-term care, such as housing, nutrition, and transportation, are services that all of us consume daily but become an integral part of long-term care for a person with a disability. Disabilities can affect housing needs, nutritional needs, or transportation needs. But, what is more important is that where one wants to live or what activities one wants to pursue also affects how needed services can be provided. Providing personal assistance in a congregate setting such as a nursing home or assisted living facility may satisfy more of an individual's needs, be more efficient, and involve more direct supervision to ensure better quality than when caregivers travel to individuals' homes to serve them one on one. Yet, those options may conflict with a person's preference to live at home and maintain autonomy in determining his or her daily activities.

REFERENCES

1. Based on our analysis of data from the Office of the Actuary of the Centers for Medicare and Medicaid Services and The MEDSTAT Group. These figures include long-term care for all people, regardless of age. Amounts do not include expenditures for nursing home and home health services provided by hospital-based entities, which are counted generally with other hospital services.

2. Through Medicaid home-and community-based services, states cover a wide variety of nonmedical and social services and supports that allow people to remain in the community. These services include personal care, personal call devices, homemakers' assistance, chore assistance, adult day health care and other services that are demonstrated as cost-effective and necessary to avoid institutionalization. In their home- and community-based services programs, however, states often limit eligibility or the scope of services in order to control costs.

3. Private long-term care insurance commonly includes policies that provide coverage for at least 12 months of necessary services—as demonstrated by an inability to perform a certain number of personal functions or activities of daily living—provided in settings other than acute-care hospital units.

4. For additional discussion of our long-term simulations, see U.S. General Accounting Office, Budget Issues: Long-Term Fiscal Challenges, GAO-02-467T (Washington, D.C.: February 27, 2002).

5. The specific ratios for the programs differ because of differences in the respective covered populations. Specifically, for Social Security, the ratio of covered workers to beneficiaries in 2000 was 3.4. Under the 2001 Trustees' intermediate estimates, this ratio is projected to decline to 2.1 by 2030. For Medicare Hospital Insurance, the ratio was 4.0

in 2001 and was projected to decline to 2.3 by 2030 under the 2001 Trustees' intermediate estimates.

6. Vernon Smith and Eileen Ellis, "Medicaid Budgets Under Stress: Survey Findings for State Fiscal Year 2000, 2001 and 2002," prepared for The Kaiser Commission on Medicaid and the Uninsured (Washington, D.C.: The Henry J. Kaiser Family Foundation, Oct. 2001).

7. Judith Feder et al., "Long-Term Care in the United States: An Overview," Health Affairs, May/June 2000, pp. 40 to 56.

8. "Aging into the 21st Century," prepared by Jacob Siegel for the Administration on Aging, U.S. Department of Health and Human Services, May 1996.

9. Assistant Secretary for Planning and Evaluation (ASPE) of the U.S. Department of Health and Human Services, who contracted with The Lewin Group, as published in Urban Institute, "Long-Term Care: Consumers, Providers, and Financing, A Chart Book" (Washington, D.C.: March 2001).

10. Data from the Medical Expenditure Panel Survey show that the average annual expenditures for home health care for all elderly individuals was $6,041 in 1996 compared to average annual expenditures for nursing home care of $20,116 for those 65 to 69 years and $25,765 for those 90 years and older.

11. Kenneth Manton and XiLiang Gu, "Changes in the Prevalence of Chronic Disability in the United States Black and Nonblack Population Above Age 65 from 1982 to 1999," Proceedings of the National Academy of Sciences of the United States of America, May 22, 2001, pp. 6354 to 6359.

12. U.S. General Accounting Office, Long-Term Care: Baby Boom Generation Increases Challenge of Financing Needed Services, GAO-01-563T (Washington, D.C.: Mar. 27, 2001) and Long-Term Care Insurance: Better Information Critical to Prospective Purchasers, GAO/T-HEHS-00-196 (Washington, D.C.: Sept. 13, 2000).

Appendix 8

The Truth about America's Healthcare System—Most Expensive Bad Results

WHAT CANNOT BE SAID ON TELEVISION ABOUT HEALTH CARE[*]

Ezekiel J. Emanuel, MD, PhD

"BEST HEALTH CARE SYSTEM IN THE WORLD"

It used to be an accepted trope for US politicians to puff up their chests and pronounce that the United States had the best health care system in the world. Simultaneously, they would vehemently denounce as unpatriotic anyone who hinted that there were serious problems with the US health care system. In 2001, while testifying to a House subcommittee, I personally experienced a congressman's wrath when I noted that many Americans with colorectal cancer were not getting appropriate adjuvant chemotherapy. Incredulous, he demanded to know if "God forbid, you should ever have cancer, where [besides the United States] would you choose to be treated?"[1] Politicians could say such things because Americans believed them. Even if people somehow knew there were problems, there was a sense that the United States had the best—that those who were rich and could afford anything or were admitted to one of America's great teaching hospitals were getting the best health care available anywhere in the world. This is no longer true. Many no longer believe the United States has the best health care system in the world.[2] The statistics are damning. The United States has the most expensive system, by far. In 2005 health care cost more than $6000 per person or in excess of 16% of the gross domestic product (GDP).[3] The nearest rival, Switzerland, spends $4077 per person per year, or 11.5% of its GDP (in purchasing power parity).[4] Norway spends $3966 (9.7% of GDP); Germany, $3043 (10.6% of GDP); and South Korea, a mere $1149 (8.2% of GDP).[5] However, Americans are increasingly aware that all of this money is not buying very much. Life expectancy in the United

[*]What Cannot Be Said on Television About Health Care *Journal of the American Medical Association*, May 16, 2007. Vol. 297, No. 19: 2131–2133 (PMID 17507349). Copyright © 2007, American Medical Association. All rights reserved. Used with permission.

States is 78 years, ranking 45th in the world, well behind Switzerland, Norway, Germany, and even Greece, Bosnia, and Jordan.[6] The US infant mortality rate is 6.37 per 1000 live births, higher than almost all other developed countries, as well as Cuba. Even for white individuals, the numbers are not world class—5.7 infant deaths per 1000 live births—more than double the rate in Singapore, Sweden, and Japan.[7] Even at the individual hospital level, Americans are realizing the care they receive is not of the highest quality.

• • •

Within the last few years, the tipping point has been passed. Something has radically changed when the *New Yorker* claims the system is a mess[8] and when United Healthcare, a corporate pillar of the status quo, opens an advertisement in the *Wall Street Journal* by boldly stating that "The health system isn't healthy. There's no denying it. A system that was designed to make you feel better often just makes things worse."[9] The US health care system is considered a dysfunctional mess. Conventional wisdom has been turned on its head. If a politician declares that the United States has the best health care system in the world today, he or she looks clueless rather than patriotic or authoritative.

• • •

The tipping point came when the media began reporting that the high cost of pharmaceuticals forced some elderly to choose between drugs and food.[10] Health care actually was being traded off against other goods both at the individual and social level. The implication was that for Americans, health care did not necessarily seem so special; other essential needs—food, housing, or heating—could be just as special. The same phenomenon began to play out in state budgets. Increasing costs of Medicaid and health insurance premiums for state workers meant cuts in Medicaid's discretionary services or, more commonly, in other state services, especially primary and secondary education and support for state colleges and universities.[11]

• • •

Today, saying that health care is so special that its cost is irrelevant serves to discredit the source. A *New York Times* reporter learned this lesson the hard way when he praised a study that claimed by "virtually any commonly cited value of a year of life, we found that if medical care accounts for about half the [6.97 year] gain in life expectancy [since 1960] then the increased spending has, on average, been worth it."[12] In response, the reporter "received about 500 e-mail responses from readers, and the most common reaction was a version of a simple question: 'Why do Americans spend so much more than folks in most other developed countries while getting worse results?' "[13]

Replacing the notion that cost is irrelevant is the notion of value. Just as consumers ask whether a car or a computer is worth the cost, health care consumers are beginning to ask whether a health care intervention is worth the cost. Increasingly, health care needs to be measured by the same metrics as other goods and services—cost, quality, benefits, and value. It can no longer claim to be treated differently from other social goods.

"NEW IS BETTER"

Americans are enamored with technology, especially health technology. The US Food and Drug Administration has been urged to use surrogate markers to approve drugs and medical devices faster so they can help sick patients. Not only is the United States an early adopter of new health care technologies, many physicians are early "proliferators" of technological innovations. As shown with drug-eluting stents, physicians not only rapidly used these devices for patients who fit the clinical indications for which stents were shown to be clinically beneficial, but nearly 60% of stents were implemented for off-label indications, ie, use in patients with lesions for which the stents have not been shown in clinical trials to be beneficial.[14] Similarly, approximately 1 in 7 prescriptions is for off-label use of drugs not supported by published evidence.[15]

Author Affiliation: Department of Clinical Bioethics, The Clinical Center, National Institutes of Health, Bethesda, Md. Corresponding Author: Ezekiel J. Emanuel, MD, PhD, Department of Clinical Bioethics, National Institutes of Health, Bldg 10 Room 1C118, Bethesda, MD 208921156 (eemanuel@nih.gov).

REFERENCES

1. Committee on Energy and Commerce; Subcommittee on Oversight and Investigations. Medicare drug reimbursements: a broken system for patients and taxpayers. September 21, 2001. http://frwebgate.access.gpo.gov/cgi-bin/getdoc.cgi?dbname=107_house_hearings&docid=f:75756.wais. Accessed April 25, 2007.

2. Schoen C, Blendon RJ, DesRoches CM, Osborn R. Comparison of health care system views and experiences in five nations, 2001: findings from the Commonwealth Fund 2001 international health policy survey. Issue Brief. May 2002.

3. Catlin A, Cowan C, Heffler S, Washington B; National Health Exenditures Accounts Team. National health spending in 2005: the slowdown continues. Health Aff (Millwood). 2007;26:142–153.

4. Organisation for Economic Co-operation and Development. OECD Health Data 2006: Statistics and Indicators for 30 Countries. http://www.oecd.org/document /16/0,2340,en_2649_34631_2085200_1_1_1_1,00.html. Accessed April 25, 2007.

5. Ibid.

6. Central Intelligence Agency. The World Factbook. https://www.cia.gov/cia /publications/factbook/rankorder/2102rank.html. Accessibility verified April 23, 2007.

7. Organisation for Economic Co-operation and Development. OECD Health Data 2006: Statistics and Indicators for 30 Countries. http://www.oecd.org/document /16/0,2340,en_2649_34631_2085200_1_1_1_1,00.html. Accessed April 25, 2007.

8. Hertzberg H. Consumption. New Yorker. April 17, 2006. http://www.newyorker .com/archive/2006/04/17/060417ta_talk_hertzberg. Accessed April 26, 2007.

9. United Healthcare. Advertisement. Wall Street Journal. March 19, 2007:A5.

10. Carey J. Commentary: costly drugs: an even bloodier backlash ahead. Business-Week Online. May 28, 2001. http://www.businessweek.com/magazine/content/01_22/b3734079.htm. Accessibility verified April 25, 2007.

11. Fossett JW, Burke CE. Medicaid and State Budgets in FY 2004: Why Medicaid Is So Hard to Cut. Albany, N.Y.: Rockefeller Institute of Government; July 2004. http://www.rockinst.org/publications/federalism/medicaid_managed_care/MedicaidandStateBudgets2004.pdf.

12. Cutler DM, Rosen AB, Vijan S. The value of medical spending in the United States, 1960–2000. N Engl J Med. 2006;355:920–927.

13. Leonhardt D. A lesson from Europe on health care. New York Times. October 18, 2006:D1.

14. Shuchman M. Debating the risks of drug eluting stents. N Engl J Med. 2007; 356:325–328.

15. Radley DC, Finkelstein SN, Stafford RS. Off-label prescribing among office-based physicians. Arch Intern Med. 2006;166:1021–1026.

Appendix 9

Dying in America

NATIONAL INSTITUTES OF HEALTH STATE-OF-THE-SCIENCE CONFERENCE STATEMENT ON IMPROVING END-OF-LIFE CARE[*]

NIH Consensus and State-of-the-Science statements are prepared by independent panels of health professionals and public representatives on the basis of (1) the results of a systematic literature review prepared under contract with the Agency for Healthcare Research and Quality (AHRQ), (2) presentations by investigators working in areas relevant to the conference questions during a 2-day public session, (3) questions and statements from conference attendees during open discussion periods that are part of the public session, and (4) closed deliberations by the panel during the remainder of the second day and morning of the third. This statement is an independent report of the panel and is not a policy statement of the NIH or the Federal Government. The statement reflects the panel's assessment of medical knowledge available at the time the statement was written. Thus, it provides a "snapshot in time" of the state of knowledge on the conference topic. When reading the statement, keep in mind that new knowledge is inevitably accumulating through medical research, and that the information provided is not a substitute for professional medical care or advice.

INTRODUCTION

Improvements in medical science and health care have gradually changed the nature of dying. Death is no longer predominately likely to be the sudden result of infection or injury but is now more likely to occur slowly, in old age, and at the end of a period of life-limiting or chronic illness. As a result, a demographic shift is beginning to occur that will include an increase in the number of seriously ill

[*]National Institutes of Health State-of-the-Science Conference Statement. See consensus.nih.gov/2004/2004EndOfLifeCareSOS024html.htm. December 6–8, 2004.

and dying people at the same time that the relative number of caregivers decreases. To meet this challenge, the best evidence that science can offer must be applied to guarantee the quality of care provided to the dying individual and their surviving loved ones.

The 1997 publication of the Institute of Medicine report "Approaching Death: Improving Care at the End of Life" triggered a series of activities to improve the quality of care and the quality of life at the end of life. Notable among these activities, the National Institute of Nursing Research (NINR), part of the National Institutes of Health (NIH), began a series of research solicitations that focused on issues related to end of life. Topics of the NIH initiatives have included: the clinical management of symptoms at the end of life; patterns of communication among patients, families, and providers; ethics and health care decision-making; caregiver support; the context of care delivery; complementary and alternative medicine at the end of life; dying children of all ages and their families; and informal care-giving. Research initiatives by the Robert Wood Johnson and Soros Foundations have also advanced the field.

To examine the results of these many efforts and to evaluate the current state of the science regarding care at the end of life and to identify directions for future research, the NIH convened a State-of-the-Science Conference on Improving End-of-Life Care. The conference was held on December 6–8, 2004, at the NIH in Bethesda, Maryland.

The NINR and the Office of Medical Applications of Research (OMAR) of the NIH were the primary sponsors of this meeting. The Centers for Disease Control and Prevention, the Centers for Medicare & Medicaid Services, the National Cancer Institute, the National Center for Complementary and Alternative Medicine, the National Institute of Mental Health, and the National Institute on Aging were the cosponsors.

The AHRQ supported the NIH State-of-the-Science Conference on Improving End-of-Life Care through its Evidence-based Practice Center program. Under contract to the AHRQ, the RAND Corporation and its partner, Veterans Administration Greater Los Angeles Healthcare System, developed the systematic review and analysis that served as important background for discussion at the conference.

During the first day-and-a-half of the conference, experts presented the latest end-of-life research findings to an independent panel. After weighing all of the scientific evidence, the panel drafted a statement addressing the following key questions:

1. What defines the transition to end of life?
2. What outcome variables are important indicators of the quality of the end-of-life experience for the dying person and for the surviving loved ones?
3. What patient, family, and health care system factors are associated with improved or worsened outcomes?
4. What processes and interventions are associated with improved or worsened outcomes?
5. What are the future research directions for improving end-of-life care?

On the final day of the conference, the panel chairperson read the draft statement to the conference audience and invited comments and questions. A press conference followed to allow the panel to respond to questions from the media.

1. WHAT DEFINES THE TRANSITION TO END OF LIFE?

The evidence does not support a precise definition of the interval referred to as end of life or its transitions. End of life is usually defined and limited by the regulatory environment rather than by the scientific data. A regulatory definition is a barrier to improving care and research relating to end of life. End of life should not be defined by a specific timeframe unless evidence can support reliable prognostication.

There are individuals for whom identification of end of life is relatively clear; however, data support that this is relatively uncommon. The data demonstrate that it is not possible to accurately predict an individual's time of death.

There has been a lack of definitional clarity related to several concepts and terms, such as palliative care, end-of-life care, and hospice care. Too often these terms are used interchangeably and the distinctions for each term must be clarified to patients and their families, providers, policymakers, and investigators. The lack of definition for the key terms represents a barrier to research in improving end-of-life care. There is insufficient evidence to determine what differences exist in the definitions of the end-of-life experience based upon gender, race, region, or ethnicity.

Respect for choice (patient or proxy), especially at the end of life, is a central value. However, patient and provider expectations and/or the desire for resource-intensive therapies with a small chance of benefit may clash with societal priorities.

Components of End of Life

There is no exact definition of end of life; however, the evidence supports the following components: (1) the presence of a chronic disease(s) or symptoms or functional impairments that persist but may also fluctuate; and (2) the symptoms or impairments resulting from the underlying irreversible disease require formal (paid, professional) or informal (unpaid) care and can lead to death. Older age and frailty may be surrogates for life-threatening illness and comorbidity; however, there is insufficient evidence for understanding these variables as components of end of life.

Transitions to End of Life

Life is a continuum and individuals traverse this continuum facing illnesses and limited functionality. Evidence does not support defining end of life as crossing an arbitrary threshold. Administrative thresholds may be justifiable but should be based on solid science. The end-of-life process includes numerous transitions: physical, emotional, spiritual, and financial. There are also transitions in health care systems exacerbated by the lack of continuity among caregivers, challenges to social support networks, unshared clinical information, and multiple physical locations for care. Family members experience role transitions, stress, and, ultimately, bereavement as their loved one traverses life's continuum. Family and professional caregivers face similar challenges as well.

2. WHAT OUTCOME VARIABLES ARE IMPORTANT INDICATORS OF THE QUALITY OF THE END-OF-LIFE EXPERIENCE FOR THE DYING PERSON AND FOR THE SURVIVING LOVED ONES?

The outcome domains and measured variables for the end-of-life experience have been described in several documents: "Describing Death in America, What We Need to Know" (prepared by the Institute of Medicine), "Clinical Practice Guidelines for Quality Palliative Care" (prepared by the National Consensus Project for Quality Palliative Care), and "End-of-Life Care and Outcomes" (prepared by Southern California Evidence-based Practice Center RAND Corporation) as well as expert testimony and public comment presented to the panel.

Examples of broad outcome domains related to end of life include physical or psychological symptoms, social relationships, spiritual or philosophical beliefs, hopes, expectations and meaning, satisfaction, economic considerations, and caregiver and family experiences. Quality of life is a domain commonly proposed as an end-of-life outcome.

However, the association between quality of life and end-of-life care could be strengthened by clear definitions and consistent measurements of quality of life.

The outcome domains are influenced by structure and process variables. Examples of structural variables of care include settings, provider education, demographics, geography, information systems, political systems, policies, regulations, and finances. Examples of processes of care domains include disease, syndrome and symptom management, continuity, goals and plans, monitoring and quality management, decisionmaking, and communication.

Summary of Measurement Issues

Based on the evidence:

1. Valid measures exist, as applied to some aspects of end of life, among individuals with cancer. However, these same measures have not been used consistently or validated longitudinally in other diseases or in diverse settings or with diverse groups.
2. Proxies, defined as surrogate responders for persons at end of life, are frequently the only source of measurement for an end-of-life outcome.
3. The evidence indicates that proxies report objective states, such as mobility, more accurately than they report subjective states, such as pain, depression, or fatigue.

4. Missing data are a limitation of most measures when used in persons at the end of life. Many measures may not be of use among persons with severe cognitive and/or communication disorders.
5. There are insufficient measures for evaluating end-of-life outcomes among children and their caregivers.
6. Few tools have undergone rigorous examination for conceptual and measurement equivalence among groups sampled from ethnically diverse populations.

3. WHAT PATIENT, FAMILY, AND HEALTH CARE SYSTEM FACTORS ARE ASSOCIATED WITH IMPROVED OR WORSENED OUTCOMES?

In general, research on the patient, family, and system factors that improve or worsen outcomes is limited. The research that has been conducted has used small samples and studies of narrowly defined populations. Thus, the results may not be applicable to larger groups or patients with diverse racial and ethnic backgrounds. Among the most important factors to be considered are: race, culture and ethnicity, socioeconomic status, sexual orientation, disease states, age, settings of care, and level of disability. All require further study.

Although race, culture, and ethnicity are difficult to define, they are associated with disparities in access to health care, quality of health care delivery, and health care outcomes. The reasons for these disparities are multiple, including provider factors (stereotyping and provider bias), patient factors (different values, attitudes, beliefs, and preferences in end-of-life care), and other health care system factors (inadequate translation and interpreter services). Disparities have been shown in the treatment of pain and symptom management in end-of-life care. Some minority groups have shown a preference for more intense therapy rather than hospice at the end of life. Additionally, minorities are underrepresented in end-of-life research.

Disease state can also affect end-of-life care. Whether one has cancer, heart disease, or dementia affects the pattern of functional decline, ability to interact with health care providers, attitudes of health care providers and caregivers, and manifestation of symptoms. Most of the end-of-life research has been done in patients with specific single disease states, such as cancer, and to a lesser extent in dementia. Moreover, the sickest patients and those with comorbidities are often excluded from research studies.

Assessment and management of symptoms have been most thoroughly studied in patients with cancer. However, other life-limiting illnesses, such as congestive heart failure, end-stage renal disease, chronic obstructive pulmonary disease, liver failure, and dementia, present their own unique challenges in end-of-life care. For example, in the case of dementia, providers often do not recognize dementia as a terminal illness. Communication is more complex, often due to cognitive deficits and the need for surrogate decisionmakers. Tools for measuring end-of-life care and to evaluate outcomes have not been validated in patients with dementia.

Setting of care, level of disability, and age are other factors that influence outcomes in end-of-life care and bereavement. The level of training of staff varies across settings and types of care (e.g., nursing homes, community hospitals, university hospitals, and hospice). The most functionally disabled patients require substantial support for basic activities of daily living. Of special note, there is a dearth of evidence on end-of-life treatment of children. The evidence comes from small, single site studies. What evidence there is suggests that fear of being forgotten, fear of pain, and fear of causing family sorrow, while common across patients of all ages, may represent unique challenges for children and their families. Recent reviews show that there are no instruments available for measuring the end-of-life experience in children. Due to this lack of data, it is difficult to draw broad conclusions. Researching the end-of-life experience in children and adults is complicated by the fact that institutional review boards are especially sensitive to the distress of the dying children and their families as well as to other vulnerable populations and, therefore, are reluctant to approve such studies.

General system factors can also affect outcomes. At the health care system level, one of the biggest problems noted is that care is fragmented, consisting of multiple providers, and requires the patients to make many transitions in their care. Other problems include lack of flow of information across providers and settings as well as different skill levels of providers and financial incentives that perpetuate discontinuity and discourage high-quality care.

Research is needed to create and evaluate models of care. Some models of effective integrated care at the end of life have been developed, usually in academic settings or in closed health care systems (most notably within the veterans health care system). They have not been applied or evaluated in the settings where most persons at the end of life receive their care.

The design of the current Medicare hospice benefit limits the availability of the full range of interventions needed by many persons at the end of life. These design limits include, for example, a 6-month prognostication to death; a forced choice between skilled care and hospice care for Medicare patients entering nursing homes from hospitals; limitations on the availability of therapies, such as radiation for symptom management; and requirements for "pass through" payments between hospice and nursing home providers. Furthermore, although hospice has been a leader in the evolution of end-of-life care, the research on the hospice program is limited. The two randomized studies were conducted more than 20 years ago. More recent observational studies suffer from selection bias because they are limited to those who have chosen the hospice benefit.

Attention must also be paid to how State Medicaid policy affects end-of-life care for the significant number of patients who are "dually eligible" for Medicare and Medicaid. In theory, this creates the potential for integrated care (as demonstrated in PACE—the Program for All-Inclusive Care for the Elderly). There is evidence that state policy often creates barriers to care that need to be identified and addressed.

4. WHAT PROCESSES AND INTERVENTIONS ARE ASSOCIATED WITH IMPROVED OR WORSENED OUTCOMES?

There is a growing body of research related to specific care interventions designed to improve outcomes for the end-of-life experience for patients and families. These include interventions in symptom management, spiritual aspects of dying, withdrawal of life-sustaining treatments, family caregiving, and bereavement. Effective communication is critical to the success of these interventions.

The following findings from these studies are of note.

- The quality of evidence on symptom management appears to be limited, with the exception of pain management. Although considerable research has been done regarding the use of medications in the management of pain, these protocols have not been widely incorporated into practice. While specific end-of-life curricula have been developed, they are being used inconsistently to train health care professionals. They have not been evaluated and the outcome of the training is not known. Conclusions regarding the benefits of symptom management with complementary and alternative medicine suffer from insufficient numbers of studies, small samples, and weak study designs.
- Studies in the area of bereavement interventions indicate that, for some groups of adults, interventions are most effective when requested by the grieving party. More studies are needed to evaluate the more complicated forms of grief, especially in particularly vulnerable populations, including grieving children.
- Encouragement to initiate advance directives (i.e., legal documents, such as living wills and health care powers of attorney) alone have not been shown to improve outcomes among individuals with diseases other than dementia; however, the reasons for this are not well-known. Little evidence of the effect of advance directives on care of people with impaired decisionmaking ability was presented. Advanced-care planning—a process for preparing for the end of life, including discussion of death— is different from advanced directives and needs further study to examine its effectiveness.
- Communication among providers, patients, and families is believed to improve care. Communication is important as the common pathway to the relief of suffering; it generates gratitude and complaints and is an important component of palliative care. Some studies have shown improvement in communication skills of providers. Others have shown that physicians and nurses sometimes underestimate or do not elicit the full range of patient concerns and do not show empathy. A majority of the studies on interventions to enhance communication have been done outside the United States in small samples, which yielded intriguing results. It is not known how these will translate into the U.S. population.

- Effective multidisciplinary communication may be particularly important in the case of children where parents are the primary decision-makers. In particular, the absence of realistic hope with regard to pain and suffering has been shown to diminish the responsiveness of parents to initiating end-of-life discussions.
- Spirituality is consistently defined as a critical domain in end-of-life care; research on interventions to improve spiritual wellbeing is very limited. Preliminary evidence of a specific intervention—dignity therapy—shows positive outcomes for both the patient and family in terms of satisfaction and heightened sense of dignity, purpose, meaning, and grief management.
- Research on withholding and withdrawing life-sustaining treatment has been conducted most often in the intensive-care setting.
- Family caregivers are central to end-of-life care because they provide emotional support and essential help with activities of daily living, medications, and eating as well as communicate with health care professionals. Although both educational and supportive interventions have been tested, only a limited number of randomized clinical trials have been conducted with caregivers of patients near end of life. There is limited information, aside from dementia, and little information about culturally diverse populations. However, there is a lack of data regarding which caregivers are at greatest risk for distress and which interventions are likely to relieve that distress. Little evidence was provided regarding the experiences of professional caregivers at the end of life. There is a need to examine their experiences and projections regarding future availability.

In spite of the many studies that have evaluated these and other interventions, as a body of intervention research on enhancing the end-of-life experience for patients and families, this work has several limitations that warrant further consideration in future research:

1. Most interventions tested are either not theory-based, or the theories they are based on are not stated explicitly.
2. Details of interventions are not always available in publications of results or in protocol manuals that are publicly available. As a result, these interventions cannot be replicated, improved, or tested in other care settings.
3. Most interventions include multiple components, with limited attention given to the conditions under which each is used. As a result, care to those receiving these interventions is not always provided in the same way and separate components of multi-component interventions cannot be evaluated so that programs can be improved.
4. Fidelity to components of multi-component interventions is not typically examined; as a result, it is not known how different component interventions are used and by which groups of patients and providers.

5. Many of the studies are limited to small numbers of patients in select care settings and in select patient populations, thereby limiting generalizability and restricting the ability to demonstrate null effects.

6. Many studies either do not rely on randomized designs or do not include comparison groups, which limits the ability to draw conclusions about the effect of the treatment versus the usual outcome course.

7. Many different outcome measures have been used. While not necessarily a limitation for any single study, the use of a diverse set of outcome measures limits the ability to draw comparisons across studies of the same or different interventions.

8. Few of the intervention studies include assessments of costs to patients, families, or the health care system; and few studies evaluate the cost-effectiveness of interventions. Without these assessments, it will be difficult to judge the extent to which they can be implemented in real-world contexts now or in the future.

5. WHAT ARE FUTURE RESEARCH DIRECTIONS FOR IMPROVING END-OF-LIFE CARE?

End-of-life care has emerged as a field of scientific inquiry in the past two decades. It is a vitally important area to public health in terms of resource considerations and to individuals. All people will die. Most deaths are not sudden. Most persons will experience death also as caregivers or family.

While there is a growing body of research covering a wide range of issues, the research is, in many ways, still in its infancy in terms of rigorous testing and evaluation of models of care, in terms of patients and family outcomes, and in terms of resource utilization. Research is needed to understand patient, caregiver, and health care system influences on these outcomes.

Conceptual Models

- Develop conceptual models/frameworks to guide the full range (qualitative and quantitative, descriptive, and randomized-controlled trials) of systematic research in end-of-life care as it affects patients, families, and care providers. This would include providing operational definitions of end-of-life and palliative care.
- Efforts should be made for further development and consensus about common definitions and constructs as they relate to end-of-life and palliative care.

Infrastructure

- Create a network of end-of-life investigators and well-defined cohorts of patients to facilitate coordinated interdisciplinary, multisite studies. This should include establishing new networks of end-of-life investigators as well as expanding existing networks (such as the National Clinical Trials Cooperative Groups) so they have a critical mass of end-of-life investigators and appropriate study populations. These networks should enhance training of a new generation of interdisciplinary scientists (through funding mechanisms, such as K-awards, T32s, and R25s).

Methodologic Issues

- Develop a consensus regarding a minimum set of measures that can be used to assess end-of-life domains in well-defined cohort studies established at multisites.
- Categorize measures in terms of several factors, including source of information (e.g., patient, family, staff), level of information (e.g., self-report, observational rating, physiological), cognitive requirements (e.g., can be obtained from communication impaired, level of cognitive capacity required), and validation samples (e.g., was validated among minority groups).
- Measurement tools require testing for equivalence, validity, and sensitivity to change within and across well-defined disease, racial, ethnic, age, gender, and cultural groups.
- Determine and seek to improve the reliability and validity of data obtained from proxies as they vary by rater, relationship, domain, and over time.
- Develop and utilize instruments with an awareness of minimizing burdens on patients near end of life and their families.

Ethical Issues

- Attend to normative ethical questions regarding such things as the concept of a good death, and identify and resolve ethical problems in end-of-life care that arise from conflicting needs of caregivers and care receivers.
- Explore ethical issues in end-of-life research pertinent to institutional review boards, ethics committees, and study sections to reduce barriers to conducting research without compromising ethical standards.

Treatment

- Develop and test new interventions in diverse patient groups with a variety of primary and co-morbid conditions to improve the end-of-life experience for patients and their loved ones.
- Develop and test new interventions, including complementary and alternative medicines, to improve symptom management in diverse patient groups.
- Design studies to enlist patients and families starting at the beginning of a serious illness in order to capture transitions and end-of-life trajectories. (One strategy might be to piggy-back onto longitudinal studies to include measures that would capture the end-of-life trajectory through bereavement.)

- Determine how individual, family, and health care system factors affect responses to care in home, hospice, long-term, and acute care settings.
- Study effective communication and documentation of components of end-of-life discussions in advanced-care planning.
- Develop and evaluate strategies for translating efficacious interventions to enhance end-of-life care into practice in a broad array of real-world settings, and evaluate the cost and effectiveness of these interventions through rigorously designed research.
- Increase knowledge related to patient preferences for information and establish a strong link with specific communication behaviors and outcomes. Identify strategies to enhance care provider communication skills surrounding end of life.

Outcomes

- Studies should be attentive to the recruitment of underrepresented populations, and the studies should be adequately powered to evaluate well-defined subgroup (e.g., disease, race, ethnicity, age, region, gender) differences. This will likely require multicenter studies. The creation of end-of-life research networks will facilitate representative samples along with larger sample size, encourage uniformity in measures, and increase interdisciplinary collaboration.
- Intervention trials for patients at end of life should include some focus on family caregivers, especially in cases such as dementia and ventilator-dependent patients.
- Conduct demonstrations in and across clinical settings to evaluate the outcomes and costs of models of care delivery to determine their economic and clinical feasibility in real-world settings.
- Attention must be paid to the surviving loved ones of those who die from sudden or accidental death. Research needs to be conducted to evaluate the needs of this population.

Policy

- Increase the funding of end-of-life research within the NIH, the AHRQ, the Health Resources and Services Administration, the Department of Veterans Affairs, the Centers for Medicare & Medicaid Service, the Department of Health and Human Services, and the Centers for Disease Control and Prevention.
- Encourage interinstitute and interagency coordination and funding of end-of-life research. End of life is pertinent to most patient populations, including such diverse populations as children and people with end-stage organ failure, including heart, lung, and kidney, as well as those with cancer, dementia, psychiatric disabilities, and addictions.
- Explore public–private partnerships related to end-of-life research support.

- Develop, test, and evaluate new models of end-of-life care for Medicare beneficiaries designed to overcome identified limitations of and barriers to utilization of the current Medicare hospice benefit.
- Conduct studies of State Medicaid policy to identify barriers to and financial disincentives for effective end-of-life care.
- Increase Federal funding to enhance health care provider knowledge related to end-of-life research to ensure the timely translation of research findings to clinical practice.
- Develop and use retrospective data from representative samples of Americans on the health, quality of life and care, and use of health care resources in the period preceding death. To further develop and enhance capabilities in this area, we endorse the recommendations of the 2003 Institute of Medicine report "Describing Death in America," which calls for support of researchers' use of existing data systems, improving the use of existing data systems, and conduct of a new National Mortality Followback Survey.

CONCLUSIONS

- Circumstances surrounding end of life are poorly understood, leaving many Americans to struggle through this life event.
- The dramatic increase in the number of older adults facing the need for end-of-life care warrants development of a research infrastructure and resources to enhance that care for patients and their families.
- Ambiguity surrounding the definition of end-of-life hinders the development of science, delivery of care, and communications between patients and providers.
- Current end-of-life care includes some untested interventions that need to be validated.
- Subgroups of race, ethnicity, culture, gender, age, and disease states experience end-of-life care differently, and these differences remain poorly understood.
- Valid measures exist for some aspects of end of life; however, measures have not been used consistently or validated in diverse settings or with diverse groups.
- End-of-life care is often fragmented among providers and provider settings, leading to a lack of continuity of care and impeding the ability to provide high-quality, interdisciplinary care.
- Enhanced communication among patients, families, and providers is crucial to high-quality end-of-life care.
- The design of the current Medicare hospice benefit limits the availability of the full range of interventions needed by many persons at the end of life.

STATE-OF-THE-SCIENCE PANEL

A complete list of the participants in this panel may be found at http://consensus. nih.gov/2004/2004EndOfLifeCareSOS024html.htm.

Appendix 10

Universal Healthcare in America: The Lure of a Quick Fix

Kenneth A. Fisher, M. D.

Universal healthcare is a hot topic right now. Political leaders talk of the need for it and make half-hearted attempts to come up with some plan or other that just doesn't fly. Pundits bemoan the shame of the world's richest country having no universal healthcare, and over 46 million people are without any kind of health insurance at all. To top it off, we spend much more per person on healthcare than any other nation, but we have higher infant mortality and a lower disease-adjusted life expectancy.

So why don't we have universal health coverage? Why do millions of Americans use the overly expensive emergency room as an ill-conceived place for primary care? What are the fundamental flaws in our medical system that make health-care so outrageously expensive and out of the reach of so many Americans? And, more important, how can we fix them?

We can certainly learn from other industrialized countries with universal coverage. At the same time, we must understand that we have our own unique healthcare history, a political/social culture that feels less government is best, and that we are a very large nation.

Many people hold the Canadian healthcare system up as an example of what can be done, so let's take a look at that system compared to our own.

THE CANADIAN HEALTHCARE SYSTEM

The Canadian system was initiated in 1957 with federal legislation providing monies for the provinces to establish universal hospital insurance, with physician services added in 1968. However, in 1977, the federal government decreased its commitment to fund about 50 percent of the provinces' costs, causing the provinces to alter coverage or raise their own taxes. In 1984, because of federal penalties, all provinces disallowed physicians from billing patients' additional fees above the provincial payment.

The systems in each jurisdiction are somewhat autonomous. But to obtain federal funds, the provinces and territories must have these features:

1. Provision of all medical services (hospital and physician).
2. Public administration of the system.
3. Portability throughout the country.
4. Universal coverage.
5. Absence of additional charges by physicians and hospitals.

Physicians work as independent contractors for a fixed fee for service, and hospitals, although referred to as "public," are privately owned, not-for-profit entities. Nationally, the system allows only for private insurance coverage for perks such as private rooms. As conditions change, each province has to readjust its coverages (e.g., for home-based care and pharmaceuticals) long before the federal government responds. In the 1990s, federal payments to the provinces decreased dramatically, causing many hospitals to close or merge. Some federal funding was restored in 2000, but the public perception had changed and the system was under intense political pressure, with 59 percent in 2001 feeling the system needed fundamental reform and the majority of voices calling for a larger role for private enterprise. Two high-level commissions were formed (Romanov and Kirby reports), gave their recommendations, and in 2003 the federal government agreed to significantly increase funding. Areas for which the federal government promised to increase funding were medical equipment, physician and nurse manpower needs, an electronic medical record system, better care for native Canadians, enhanced primary care, and more transparency and accountability.[1] However, there is a fair degree of skepticism that these reforms will come to fruition.

THE U.S. AND CANADIAN SYSTEMS IN CONTRAST

Until the 1950s the Canadian and American healthcare systems were similar. As recently as 1971, Canada spent 7.0 percent of gross domestic product (GDP) for healthcare while the United States spent a similar amount, 7.6 percent. Currently, the core difference between the two systems is private insurance, universal coverage, and cost. In the mid-1960s, both countries developed a government-funded health system. The United States opted for a system only for those over age sixty-five (Medicare) and for the poor (Medicaid). The remainder of the covered population is privately insured, mostly through employment. Canada adopted a universal coverage, taxpayer-funded, government-operated system.[2]

However, many services are not covered by the Canadian plan. After age fourteen, dental services are not covered, and some provinces cover optometry (eye glasses) while others do not. Visits to specialists may require a user fee, and circumcision is not covered. Two provinces, Alberta and Quebec, one with a conservative and the other a liberal government, are expanding the private sector within their healthcare system. Canadian courts have recently held that the government cannot prevent citizens from buying private insurance to augment services, not only in the private but also in the public system. Thus, there is movement in Canada to have a mixed system such as now exists in the United States.[3]

In the 1960s, when other Western democracies such as Canada were developing their publicly funded universal healthcare programs, they were living under the very expensive military umbrella of the United States in the midst of the cold war with the Soviet Union. Because they didn't have the expense of maintaining an extensive military, these countries were able to fund their healthcare programs and at the same time be secure from the Soviet military threat. Meanwhile, in the United States there were not funds to support both a much larger military and provide universal healthcare.

Because of the differential in pay and standard of living between Canadian healthcare professionals and their U.S. counterparts, many physicians leave Canada after their training is complete at the Canadian government's expense. The lure of practicing in the United States, where independence and autonomy are more possible, is irresistible to many. Although this migration has slowed in recent years, there still is a significant shortage of physicians in Canada. About 10 percent of the population does not have a physician.[4] However, this is less than the 15–16 percent of Americans without health insurance who must obtain their healthcare in emergency rooms or free clinics. (Free clinics see about 3.5 million patients annually in the United States.)

Although the costs for healthcare were similar for the two countries in the early 1970s, that certainly is no longer the case. As of 2001, the United States spent $4,887/person (almost twice that amount today[5]) while Canada spent $2,792/person.[6] Some of this difference in cost is due to:

1. More violence and drug abuse in the United States.
2. More illegal aliens who need to use expensive emergency rooms for their medical care.
3. More veterans of warfare in the United States needing healthcare because of injuries.
4. Different accounting practices in the United States and Canada, making financial comparisons difficult.
5. Fewer high-priced technologies (MRIs, CAT scanners, etc.) per capita in Canada, with patients coming to the United States for these tests. Thus Canada is using U.S. capital investments to meet these high-ticket needs.
6. A much lower per capita medical research budget in Canada versus that in the United States.
7. Higher pay for health professionals in the United States.
8. Much higher administrative costs in the U.S. health system.
9. Fewer laws in Canada like the U.S.'s Patient Self-Determination Act and the Americans with Disabilities Act, which cause confusion and chaos in end-of-life situations.

10. Less reliance on technology and procedures in Canada versus the United States, but with similar outcomes and more reliance on primary care.[7]
11. More expensive malpractice insurance in the United States.

In measures of healthcare quality, Canada has better results than the United States.

1. Life expectancy is about two and one half years less in the United States.
2. Infant and child mortality is higher in the United States.
3. Overall death rates/100,000 citizens is 8.5 deaths lower for woman and 2.3 deaths lower for men in Canada versus the United States.

Many of these differences can be accounted for by the greater diversity of the American population, which is ten times larger than that of Canada, with many more poor and disadvantaged. The American healthcare system has a unique history, a certain set of values that are less government-oriented than that of most other nations, and an incomparably large population. When others talk about implementing aspects of a system from another country, such as Canada, they ignore the facts that Canada has its own problems with its healthcare system and it is a nation of 30 million people, while we in the United States have a population of 300 million people, not to mention greater cultural, religious, and ethnic diversity. To complicate the issue, there is little agreement on just how to calculate our administrative costs and less agreement on how to fix it.

HISTORY OF ATTEMPTS FOR A NATIONAL HEALTH PLAN IN THE UNITED STATES

There have been five attempts to provide universal healthcare in the United States.[8]

1. The American Association for Labor Legislation proposed a national insurance system in 1915 that would cover medical care, sick pay, maternity, and funeral expenses. The final proposal was to cover a large segment of our society; it would be funded by employer, employee, and state monies; and it was called a social insurance plan, but it was not universal because it would cover only those who contributed to the fund. The plan was opposed by the American Medical Association (AMA), business, and labor groups and with the advent of World War I was defeated.
2. In the early 1940s, Senators Robert Wagner and James Murray, along with Representative John Dingell, proposed to expand Social Security, which came into existence in 1935, to pay for physician and hospital care for workers and retirees. Employers and employees would pay for

workers, with government and charity care for the unemployed. After World War II, in 1945, President Truman supported the plan, but the AMA fought vigorously against it and it was defeated.

3. The first national health insurance plan in the United States came into fruition in July 1965, when President Johnson signed Medicare/Medicaid into effect. Medicare, a descendant of the Wagner-Murray-Dingle bill, was different in that it was only for those 65 and older and is funded from Social Security, federal taxes, and individual premiums. Medicaid, the first public assistance health coverage, is need-based and does not require recipients to have paid into the plan. Medicare/Medicaid is not national health insurance because it does not include all citizens of the United States. Medicare and Medicaid was passed over the objections of the AMA.

4. In the 1970s, Senator Edward Kennedy and Representative Martha Griffiths proposed universal healthcare for all Americans to replace Medicare/Medicaid and be funded by employer and employee contributions, and federal taxes. The Kennedy-Griffith concept was a single-payer plan that would have replaced the private health insurance industry. President Nixon opposed it and introduced the concept that the private insurance industry would continue, employers would purchase health insurance for their employees, and the government would purchase insurance for the unemployed. President Nixon and Senator Kennedy compromised and both supported the plan, but the Watergate scandal interceded and nothing became of it.

5. During the 1992 presidential election, healthcare was again a major issue. President Clinton proposed a Nixon-type plan, but with "managed competition," large purchasing cooperatives buying insurance from a decreased number of insurance companies. The plan failed.

In the aftermath of the defeat of the Clinton healthcare plan, groups supporting government-funded national health insurance initiated and developed a new proposal which was coined the single-payer plan. It was touted as a way to save billions in administrative costs. A competing concept has also emerged: an individual-based national insurance plan where everyone would be required to purchase health insurance, with the government supplying funds for purchase by the poor. As of 2003, 44 percent of healthcare is paid by the government, 35 percent by employment-based insurance, 3 percent by individuals with private insurance, and 18 percent by out-of-pocket payments. With the advent of the Medicare drug plan, out-of-pocket expenses have decreased and government expenses have increased.

BARRIERS TO UNIVERSAL COVERAGE

Universal health care is a hot topic right now. A March 2007 poll by CBS News/New York Times shows 65 percent of those polled favor universal health coverage, and that the lack universal coverage is a bigger problem than keeping healthcare costs down.[9] Political leaders talk of the need for it and bemoan the shame of the world's richest country having no universal health care, and over 47 million people without any kind of health insurance at all. To top it off, we spend much more per person on health care than any other nation, but we have higher infant mortality, and a lower disease-adjusted life expectancy.

So why don't we have universal health coverage? Why do millions of Americans use the overly expensive emergency room as an ill-conceived place for primary care? What are the fundamental flaws in our medical system that make health care so outrageously expensive and out of the reach of so many Americans? And, more importantly, how can we fix them?

As mentioned, we have "less is more" attitude toward government here in the United States, and we spend a large amount on tests and other procedures. Moreover, our administrative costs are way out of line. Universal healthcare, though tempting, is probably out of reach—and mainly due to the problems associated with financing a universal system.

No matter how we finally work out the financing of universal healthcare, we must deal with the excessive costs of our system. As this book demonstrates, a huge component of this cost is inappropriate care of those at the end of their lives. Our technological and procedural style of medicine, with its lack of compassion for the dying, is not isolated. It is emblematic of how we practice medicine in the United States, and perhaps one of the biggest barriers to creating a universal healthcare system.

FIRST STEPS: SOLVE THE EXISTING PROBLEMS FIRST

Looking through the lens of end-of-life care, this book explained the absurdities of the way we practice medicine:

- The misinterpretation of patient autonomy that forces families to make medical decisions for which they are ill prepared, causing immeasurable suffering to those they love and the unnecessary wasting of billions of dollars.
- The financial drivers at work that place a premium on technology and procedures that are terrific when used wisely, but cause misery when used inappropriately, even while making money for doctors and hospitals. This diversion of resources greatly hinders effective and available primary care, and contributes to many of our healthcare problems.
- The documented training of young physicians to practice inappropriate end-of-life care.
- The arrogance of judges who make rulings based on what they consider legal precedent rather than seeking expert medical advice about the intricacies of the individual in question.
- The inability of Congress and state legislatures to provide a legal framework by which humane end-of-life care could be given.

- The timidity of our medical societies, which do not stand for value in the delivery of care and do not participate and inform during national debates regarding controversial medical issues.

All of this results in the squandering of billions of dollars in hopeless end-of-life situations. We lose precious funding for educating our children, training nurses to ease the severe nursing shortage, and preparing young physicians to deliver appropriate care. The high cost of insuring workers is bringing our businesses and the manufacturing sectors to their knees or driving them overseas.

Every physician I know agrees that the system is flawed and, if there is no change, it will collapse under its gross inefficiencies. Almost all the families I speak with have a horror story about a dying loved one trapped in our medical system, dying a protracted, painful, dehumanizing death.

Unless and until we address the many flaws in our healthcare system, no change in the way we pay for medical care will provide a path to universal coverage. And universal healthcare will remain a pipe dream.

NOTES

1. Detsky AS, Naylor CD. Canada's health care system—reform delayed. N Engl J Med 2003; 349: 804–810 (PMID 12930935).

2. See en.wikipedia.org?wiki/Canadian_andAmerican_health_care_systems_compared (accessed April 12, 2007).

3. Ibid.

4. Ibid.

5. See www.pnhp.org (accessed May 5, 2007).

6. Reinhardt UE, Hussey PS, Anderson GF. U.S. health spending in an international context. Why is U.S. spending so high, and can we afford it? Health Affairs 2004; 23: 10–25 (PMID 15160799).

7. Kaul P, Armstrong PW, Fu Y, Knight JD, et al. Impact of different patterns of invasive care on quality of life outcomes in patients with non-ST elevation acute coronary syndrome: results from the Gusto-11b Canada-Unites States sub study. Can J Cardiol 2004; 20: 760–766 (PMID 15229756).

8. Harrison B. A historical survey of national health movements and public opinion in the United States. JAMA 2003; 289: 1163–1164 (PMID 12622591).

9. Poll: The Politics of Health Care Most Americans Favor Universal Health Care, Give Democrats Edge on Improving System. CBS News/New York Times, March 1, 2007, see www.cbsnews.com/stories/2007/03/01/opinion/polls/main2528357.shtml (Accessed August 15, 2007).

Notes

Chapter 1

1. Field MJ, Cassel CK (ed.). 1997, "How people die: Symptoms of impending death," in *Approaching Death, Improving Care at the End of Life*, Washington, D.C.: National Academy Press, p. 45.

2. Barnato AE, McClellen MB, Kagay CR, Garber AM. Trends in inpatient treatment intensity among Medicare beneficiaries at the end-of-life. *Health Services Research* 2004; 39: 363–375 (PMID 15032959).

3. Doig CJ, Burgess E. Brain death: resolving inconsistencies in the ethical declaration of death. *Canadian Journal of Anesthesia* 2003; 50: 725–731 (PMID 12944450).

4. See en.wikipedia.org/wiki/Terri_Schiavo.

5. Rich EC, Liebow M, Srinivasan M, Wolliscroft JO, Fein O, Blaser R. Medicare financing of graduate medical education: intractable problems, elusive solutions. *Journal of General Internal Medicine* 2002; 17: 283–292 (PMID 11972725).

6. Cooke M, Irby DM, Sullivan W, Ludmerer KM. American medical education 100 years after the Flexner report. *New England Journal of Medicine* 2006; 355: 1339–1344 (PMID 17005951).

7. Reinhardt UE, Hussey PS, Anderson GF. U.S. health spending in an international context. Why is U.S. spending so high, and can we afford it. *Health Affairs* 2004; 23: 10–25 (PMID 15160799).

8. Mathers CD, Sadana R, Salomon JA, Murray CJ, Lopez AD. Healthy life expectancy in 191 countries, 1999. *Lancet* 2001; 357: 1685–1691 (PMID 11425392).

9. Mathers CD, Iburg KM, Salomon JA, Taudon A, Chatterji S, Ustun B, Murray CJ. Global patterns of healthy life expectancy in the year 2002. *BMC Public Health* 2004; 4: 66 (PMID 15619327).

10. Ibid.

11. Hussey PS, Anderson GF, Osborn R, Feek C, McLaughlin V, Millar J, Epstein A. How does the quality of care compare in five countries? *Health Affairs* 2004; 23: 89–99 (PMID 15160806).

12. Census Bureau Report, 2006. *Oldest baby boomers turn 60!*

13. Aging baby boom generation will increase demand and burden on federal and state budgets. Statement of David M. Walker, Comptroller General of the United States before the Special Committee on Aging, U.S. Senate, March 21, 2002, p. 2.

14. Hoover DR, Crystal S, Kumar R, Sambamoorthi U, Cantor JC. Medical expenditures during the last year of life: findings from the 1992-1996 Medicare Beneficiary Survey. *Health Services Research* 2002; 37: 1625–1642 (PMID 12546289).

15. Emanuel EJ, Ash A, Yu W, Gazelle G, Levinsky NG, Saynina O, McClellan M, Moskowitz M. Managed care, hospice use, site of death and medical expenditures during the last year of life. *Archives of Internal Medicine* 2002; 162: 1722–1728 (PMID 12153375).

16. Levinsky NG, Yu W, Ash A, Moskowitz M, Gazelle G, Saynina O, Emanuel EJ. Influence of age on Medicare expenditures and medical care in the last year of life. *Journal of the American Medical Association*, 2001; 286: 1349–1355 (PMID 11560540).

17. Kjellstrand CM, Kovithavongs C, Szabo E. On the success, cost and efficiency of modern medicine: an international comparison. *Journal of Internal Medicine* 1998; 243: 3–14 (PMID 9487326).

18. See www.newstarget.com/020563.html (accessed January 16, 2007).

19. See www.businessroundtable.org/pdf/LettertoPresBush_BR2006Priorities.pdf (accessed November 2006).

20. *American Medical News*, July 18, 2005.

21. Teno JM, Clarridge BR, Casey V, et al. Family perspective on end-of-life care at the last place of care. *Journal of the American Medical Association* 2004; 291: 88–93 (PMID 14709580).

22. Wood EB, Meekin SA, Fins JJ, Fleischman AR. Enhancing palliative care education in medical school curricula: implementation of palliative education assessment tool. *Academic Medicine: Journal of the Association of American Medical Colleges* 2002; 77: 285–291 (PMID 11953291).

23. Quill TE, Dannefer E, Markakis K, Epstein R, et al. An integrative biopsychological approach to palliative care training of medical students. *Journal of Palliative Medicine* 2003; 6: 365–380 (PMID 14509482).

24. Gorman TE, Ahern SP, Wiseman J, Skrobic Y. Residents end-of-life decision making with adult hospitalized patients: a review of the literature. *Academic Medicine: Journal of the Association of American Medical Colleges* 2005; 80: 622–633 (PMID 15980078).

25. Darer JD, Hwang W, Pharm HH, Bass EB, Anderson G. More training needed in chronic care: a survey of U.S. physicians. *Academic Medicine: Journal of the Association of American Medical Colleges* 2004; 79: 541–548 (PMID 15165973).

26. Feeg VD, Elebiary H. Exploratory study on end-of-life issues: barriers to palliative care and advanced directives. *American Journal of Hospice and Palliative Care* 2005; 22: 119–124 (PMID 15853089).

27. Shine KI. Geographical variation in Medicare spending (editorial). *Annals Internal Medicine* 2003; 138: 347–348 (PMID 12585834).

Chapter 2

1. *Cruzan v. Harmon*, 760 S.W.2d 408, 427 (Mo. 1989) (en banc).

2. *Cruzan*, 497 U.S. at 284.

3. See www.op.org/domcentral/study/kor/index.htm.

4. Teno J, Lynn J, Wenger N, et al. Advance directives for seriously ill hospitalized patients: effectiveness with the Patient Self Determination Act and the SUPPORT intervention. SUPPORT investigators study to understand prognoses and preferences for

outcomes and risk of treatment. *Journal of the American Geriatrics Society* 1997; 45: 500–507 (PMID 9100721).

5. Drought TS, Koenig BA. "Choice" in end-of-life decision making: researching fact or fiction. *Gerontologist* 2002; 42 Spec No. 3: 114–128 (PMID 12415142).

6. Perkins, HS. Controlling death: the false promise of advance directives. *Annals of Internal Medicine* 2007; 147: 51–57 (PMID 17606961).

7. Thomas KR. The "right to die": constitutional and statutory analysis. Congressional Research Service, p. 46, order code 97-244A. September 19, 2005.

8. Annas GJ. Asking the courts to settle standard of emergency care—the case of Baby K. *New England Journal of Medicine* 1994; 330: 1542–1545 (PMID 8164726).

9. 42 U.S.C. 1395 dd (1994) (amended 1997).

10. Angell M. The case of Helga Wanglie; a new kind of "right to die" case. *New England Journal of Medicine* 1991; 325: 511–512 (PMID 1852185).

11. Agar J. Judge rules Lawton women's life must be preserved. *Kalamazoo Gazette*, Kalamazoo, MI, April 25, 2006.

12. *American Medical News*, American Medical Association, June 12, 2006.

13. Blackhall LJ. Must we always use CPR? *New England Journal of Medicine* 1987; 317: 1281–1285 (PMID 3670350).

14. Murphy DJ, Finucane TE. New do-not-resuscitate policies. A first step in cost control. *Archives of Internal Medicine* 1993; 153: 1641–1648 (PMID 8333801).

15. Bedell SE, Delbanco TL, Cook EF, Epstein FH. Survival after cardiopulmonary resuscitation in the hospital. *New England Journal of Medicine* 1983; 309: 569–576 (PMID 6877286).

16. Taffet GE, Teasdale TA, Luchi RJ. In-hospital cardiopulmonary resuscitation. *Journal of the American Medical Association* 1988; 260: 2069–2072 (PMID 3270334).

17. Frezza EE, Squillario DM, Smith TJ. The ethical challenge and the futile treatment in the older population admitted to the intensive care unit. *American Journal of Medical Quality: The Official Journal of the American College of Medical Quality* 1998; 13: 121–126 (PMID 9735474).

18. Halpern NA, Pastores SM, Thaler HT, Greenstein RJ. Changes in critical care beds and occupancy in the United States 1985–2000: Differences attributable to hospital size. *Critical Care Medicine* 2006; 34: 2105–2112 (PMID 16755256).

19. Barnato AE, McClellan MB, Kagay CR, Garber AM. Trends in inpatient treatment intensity among Medicare beneficiaries at the end-of-life. *Health Services Research* 2004; 39: 363–375 (PMID 15032959).

20. Angus DC, Barnato AE, Linde-Zzwirble WT, et al. Use of intensive care at end of life in the United States: an epidemiologic study. *Critical Care Medicine* 2004; 32: 638–643 (PMID 15090940).

21. Esserman L, Belkora J, Lenert L. Potentially ineffective care. A new outcome to assess the limits of critical care. (Abstract-selected text). *Journal of the American Medical Association* 1995; 274: 1544–1551 (PMID 7474223). To access the full study, go to www.ncbi.nlm.nih.gov/entrez/querry. and type in the PMID number.

22. Rady MY, Johnson DJ. Admission to intensive care unit at the end-of-life: is it an informed decision? *Palliative Medicine* 2004; 18: 705–711 (PMID 15623167).

23. See en.wikipedia.org/wiki/Americans_with_Disabilities_ACT_of_1990.

24. See www.findarticles.com/p/articles/mi_m0842/is_n2_v16/ai_9373654/print.

25. See www..dhhs.gov/ocr/ada.html.

26. Lynn J. *Sick to death and not going to take it any more!* Berkeley: University of California Press, 2004.

27. Greene HL. The implantable cardioverter-defibrillator. *Clinical Cardiology* 2000; 23: 315–326 (PMID 10803438).

28. Moss AJ, Zareba W, Hall WJ, Klien H, Wilber DJ, Cannom DS, Daubert JP, Higgins SL, Brown MW, Andrews ML. Prophylactic implantation of a defibrillator in patients with myocardial infarction and reduced ejection fraction. *New England Journal of Medicine* 2002; 346: 877–883 (PMID 11907286).

29. Bigger JT. Expanding indications for implantable cardiac defibrillators (ed.). *New England Journal of Medicine* 2002; 346: 931–933 (PMID 11907294).

Chapter 3

1. Frezza EE, Squillario DM, Smith TJ. The ethical challenge and the futile treatment in the older population admitted to the intensive care unit. *American Journal of Medical Quality* 1998; 13: 121–126 (PMID 9735474).

2. Schneiderman LJ, Gilmer T, Teetzel HD, et al. Effects of ethics consultations on nonbeneficial life-sustaining treatments in the intensive care setting: a randomized controlled trial. *Journal of the American Medical Association* 2003; 290: 1166–1172 (PMID 12952998).

3. Esserman L, Belkora J, Lenert L. Potentially ineffe ctive care: A new outcome to assess the limits of critical care. *Journal of the American Medical Association* 1995; 274: 1544–1551 (PMID 7474223).

4. Cher DJ, Lenert LA. Method of Medicare reimbursement and the rate of potentially ineffective care of critically ill patients. *Journal of the American Medical Association* 1997; 278: 1001–1007 (PMID 9307348).

5. Fisher ES, Wennberg DE, Stukel TA, Gottlieb DJ, Lucus FL, Pinder EL. The implications of regional variations in Medicare spending, Parts I & II. *Annals of Internal Medicine* 2003; 138: 273–298 (PMID 12585825 and 12585826).

6. See www.cms.hhs.gov/apps/media/press/release.asp?Counter=1339 (accessed September 12, 2006).

7. MacIntyre NR, Epstein SK, Carson S, et al. Management of patients requiring prolonged mechanical ventilation: report of NAMDRC consensus conference. *Chest* 2005; 128: 3937–3954 (PMID 16354866).

8. Carson SS. Outcomes of prolonged mechanical ventilation. *Current Opinion in Critical Care* 2006; 12: 405–411 (PMID 16943717).

9. Carson SS, Bach PB, Brzozowski L, Leff A. Outcomes after long-term acute care, an analysis of 133 mechanically ventilated patients. *American Journal of Respiratory and Critical Care Medicine* 1999; 159: 1568–1572 (PMID 10228128).

10. Renal Physicians Association and American Society of Nephrology. Clinical practice guideline on shared decision-making in the appropriate initiation of and withdrawal from dialysis. Clinical Practice Guideline No. 2. Washington, D.C., November 1999; available at www.kidneyeol.org (accessed April 6, 2007).

11. Matsuyama R, Reddy S, Smith TJ. Why do patients choose chemotherapy near the end-of-life? A review of the perspective of those facing death from cancer. *Journal of Clinical Oncology* 2006; 24: 3490–3496 (PMID 16849766).

12. Medical futility in end-of-life care: report of the Council on Ethical and Judicial Affairs, AMA. *Journal of the American Medical Association* 1999; 281: 937–941 (PMID 10078492).

Chapter 4

1. Lynn J. *Sick to death and not going to take it anymore*. Berkeley: University of California Press, 2004.

2. See www.partnershipforsolutions.org (accessed December 9, 2006).

3. Anderson G, Horvath J, Knickman J, Colby D, Schear S, Jung M. *Making the case for ongoing care*. Robert Wood Foundation, available at www.partnershipforsolutions.org (accessed December 9, 2006).

4. See en.wikipedia.org/wiki/Art_Buchwald (accessed December 14, 2006).

5. See www.charter.net/news/read.php?ps=1016&id=13388849&_LT=HOME_LAR-SDCC.

6. U.S. Bureau of Labor Statistics, Monthly Labor Review. Online at www.bls.gov (accessed December 6, 2006).

7. National Council of State Boards of Nursing 2002. National council licensure examination-registered nurse/practical nurse (nclex-rn & nclex-pn) examination statistics. Statistics from years 1995–2002. Online at www.ncsbn.org/research_stats/nclex.asp (accessed December 7, 2006).

8. American Hospital Association. *2001 Trend Watch*. Online at www.aha.org (accessed December 7, 2006).

9. *End-of-Life Care: Questions and Answers*. National Cancer Institute, U.S. National Institutes of Health. October 30, 2001.

10. Ibid.

11. State Office of Communications and Public Liaison, National Institute of Neurological Disorders and Stroke. *Coma and Persistent Vegetative*. National Institutes of Health. February 2007.

12. Katz A. *Doctors say reaction of brain can be deceiving*. University of Connecticut Health Care Center, published in the *Middletown Press*, March 22, 2005.

13. Byock I. Completing the continuum of cancer care: integrating life-prolongation and palliation. *CA: A Cancer Journal for Clinicians* 2000; 50: 123–132 (PMID 10870488).

14. See www.eperc.mcw.edu (accessed December 9, 2006).

15. Ibid.

16. Finucane TE, Christmas C, Travis K. Tube feeding in patients with advanced dementia. *Journal of the American Medical Association* 1999; 282: 1365–1370 (PMID 10527184).

17. Gillick MR. Sounding board: Rethinking the role of tube feeding in patients with advanced dementia. *New England Journal of Medicine* 2000; 342: 206–210 (PMID 10639550).

18. Casarett D, Kapo J, Caplan A. Sounding board: Appropriate use of artificial nutrition and hydration—fundamental principles and recommendations. *New England Journal of Medicine* 2005; 353: 2607–2612 (PMID 16354899).

Chapter 5

1. See www.answers.com/topic/academy-of-gundishapur (accessed February 19, 2007).

2. See web.bryant.edu/~ehu/h364proj/fall_97/prier/1700-1850.html (accessed February 19, 2007).

3. See www.elderweb.com/home/book/export/html/2923 (accessed February 19, 2007). See www.med.umich.edu/1busi/history.htm (accessed February 19, 2007). See bentley.

umich.edu/bhl/BentleyMap/HTML/Text/UHospital.narrative.html (accessed February 22, 2007).

4. Fisher ES, Wennberg DE, Stukel TA, Gottlieb DJ, Lucus FL, Pinder EL. The implications of regional variations in Medicare spending, Parts I and II. *Annals of Internal Medicine* 2003; 138: 273–298 (PMID 12585825 and 12585826).

5. Cauchon D, Appleby J. Hospital building boom in burbs. *USA Today*, January 3, 2006; available at www.usatoday.com/news/health/2006-01-03-hospital-boom_x.htm (accessed November 7, 2006)

6. Bazzoli GJ, Gerland A, May J. Construction activity in U.S. hospitals: the financial impact of existing construction activity on consumers and health plans is likely to be substantial. *Health Affairs* 2006; 25: 783–791 (PMID 16684744).

7. Carpenter D. Behind the boom, What's driving hospital construction? *Trustee* 2004; 57: 6–11 (PMID 15045902).

8. Appleby J. Debate surrounds end-of-life health care costs. *USA Today*, October 18, 2006; available at www.usatoday.com/money/industries/health/2006-10-18-end-of-life-costs_x.htm (accessed December 8, 2006).

9. Romano M. Supersize me, Academic medical centers keep getting bigger, planning for future growth. *Modern Health Care* 2006; 36: 30–33 (PMID 16770967).

10. Carpenter D. Behind the boom, What's driving hospital construction? *Trustee* 2004; 57: 6–11 (PMID 15045902).

11. See en.wikipedia.org/wiki/Blue_Cross_and_Blue_Shield_Association (accessed March 8, 2007).

12. See eh.net/encyclopedia/article/thomasson.insurance.helath.us (accessed December 28, 2006).

13. Barnato AE, McClellan MB, Kagay CR, Garber AM. Trends in inpatient treatment intensity amoung Medicare beneficiaries at the end of life. *Health Services Research* 2004; 39: 363–375 (PMID 15032959).

14. Boyd DJ. The bursting state bubble and state Medicaid budgets. *Health Affairs* 2003; 22: 46–61 (PMID 12528838).

15. Vladeck BC. The political economy of Medicare. *Health Affairs* 1999; 18: 22–36 (PMID 9926643).

16. Boden WE, O'Rourke RA, Teo KK, et al. Optimal medical therapy with or without PCI for stable coronary disease. *New England Journal of Medicine* 2007; 356: 1503–1516 (PMID 17387127).

17. Woolhander S, Campbell T, Himmelstein DU. Costs of health care administration in the United States and Canada. *New England Journal of Medicine* 2003; 349: 768–775 (PMID 12930930).

18. Porter ME, Teisbert EO. How physicians can change the future of health care. *Journal of the American Medical Association* 2007; 297: 1103–1111 (PMID 17356031).

19. See www.deltahealthcare.com/pdf_files/Why-Hospitals-Buy.pdf (accessed March 2007).

20. Mechanic D. *The truth about health care: why reforms is not working on America.* New Brunswick, N.J.: Rutgers University Press, 2006.

21. Bodenheimer T, Berenson RA, Rudolf P. The primary care specialty income gap: why it matters. *Annals of Internal Medicine* 2007; 146:301-306 (PMID 17310054)

22. Ibid.

23. Kizer KW. The "new VA": a national laboratory for health care quality management. *American Journal of Medical Quality* 1999; 14: 3–20 (PMID 10446659).

24. Skinner JS, Fisher ES. Regional disparities in Medicare expenditures: an opportunity for reform. *National Tax Journal* 1997; 50: 413–425.

25. Dartmouth Atlas of Healthcare Project: See www.dartmouthatlas.org/annals/fishero3.php (accessed March 2007).

26. Report to the Congress. *Variation and innovation in Medicare*. Washington, D.C.: Medicare Payment Advisory Commission, June 2003: 8–9.

27. Fisher ES, Welch HG. Avoiding the unintended consequences of growth in medical care: how might more be worse? *Journal of the American Medical Association* 1999; 281: 446–453 (PMID 9952205).

28. Cram P, Rosenthal GE. Physician-owned specialty hospitals and coronary revascularization utilization—too much of a good thing? *Journal of the American Medical Association* 2007; 297: 998–999 (PMID 17341715).

29. Ibid.

30. *Physician-Owned Specialty Hospitals*, Report to the Congress, the Centers for Medicare and Medicaid Services and Medicare Payment Advisory Commission (MedPAC), March 2005. *Physician Owned Specialty Hospitals*, Report to U.S. Congress, U.S. Department of Health and Human Services (HHS), August 2006.

31. *Physician Owned Specialty Hospitals*, HHS Report.

32. Ferrell BR. Understanding the moral distress of nurses witnessing medically futile care. *Oncology Nursing Forum* 2006; 33: 922–930 (PMID 16955120).

33. The State of America's Hospitals—Taking the Pulse. American Hospital Association, online at www.ahapolicyforum.org/ahapolicyforum/reports.

34. U.S. Bureau of Labor Statistics. *Monthly Labor Review*. November 2005, online at www.bls.gov/opub/mlr/2005/11/art5full.pdf.

35. Health Resources and Services Administration, Aging of the Population. *Changing demographics and the implications for physicians, nurses, and other health workers*. 2003. Online at bhpr.hrsa.gov/healthworkforce/reports/changedemo/aging.htm.

36. Ibid.

37. Ibid.

38. *What is behind HRSA's projected supply, demand, and shortage of registered nurses?* Health Resources and Services Administration (HRSA). September 2004, p. 5.

39. Gosline MB. Leadership in nursing education: voices from the past. *Nursing Leadership Forum* 2004; 9: 51–59 (PMID 16033044).

40. American Hospital Association. 2001 *Trend Watch* online; online at www.aha.org (accessed December 9, 2006).

41. *What is behind HRSA's projected supply,* , pp. 10–12.

42. Bailey FA, Burgio KL, Woodby LL, Williams BR, Redden DT, Kovac SH, Durham RM, Goode PS. Improving processes of hospital care during the last hours of life. *Archives of Internal Medicine* 2005; 165: 1722–1727 (PMID 16087819).

43. Weissman DE. Decision making at a time of crisis near the end of life. *Journal of the American Medical Association* 2004; 292: 1738–1743 (PMID 15479939).

44. Fisher KA. Communicating about dying in the ICU. (Letter to the editor) *New England Journal of Medicine* 2007; 356: 2004 (PMID 17506162).

45. National Critical Care Survey, American Association of Critical-Care Nurses. *American Journal of Critical Care* January 2006.

46. Fromme EK, Bascom PB, Smith MD, Tolle SW, Hanson L, Hickam DH, Osborne ML. Survival, mortality and location of death for patients seen by a hospital-based palliative care team. *Journal of Palliative Medicine* 2006; 9: 903–911 (PMID 16910805).

Chapter 6

1. See www.pbs.org/independent/eus/almosthome/senior2.html (accessed January 7, 2007).

2. See www.pbs.org/newshour/health/nursinghomes/timeline.html (accessed February 11, 2007).

3. See en.wikipedia.org/wiki/Medicare_%28United_States%29 (accessed April 29, 2007).

4. See www.ehealthlink.com/Senior/MedicareFunding.asp (accessed April 29, 2007).

5. See en.wikipedia.org/wiki/Medicaid (accessed April 29, 2007).

6. See www.pbs.org/newshour/health/nursinghomes/facts.html (accessed March 2, 2007).

7. See www.efmoody.com/longterm/nursingstatistics.html (accessed January 19, 2007).

8. See www.agingstats.gov/chartbook2000/healthcare.html (accessed January 18, 2007).

9. See www.pbs.org/newshour/bb/health/jan-june05/mintz.html (accessed March 29, 2007).

10. See elder-law.lawers.com/Nursing-Homes.html (accessed February 9, 2007).

11. See www.boomer-books.com/nursing_homes/how-to-find-a%20nursing-home.htm (accessed February 9, 2007).

12. Spillman BC, Lubitz J. The effect of longevity on spending for acute and long-term care. *New England Journal of Medicine* 2000; 342: 1409–1415 (PMID 10805827).

13. Weil A. There's something about Medicaid: Medicaid suffers from a chronic mismatch between what we ask it to do and what we are willing to pay. *Health Affairs* 2003; 22: 13–30 (PMID 12528836).

14. Boyd DJ. The bursting state fiscal bubble and state Medicaid budgets. *Health Affairs* 2003; 22: 46–61 (PMID 12528838).

15. Zerzan J, Stearns S, Hanson L. Access to palliative care and hospice in nursing homes. *Journal of the American Medical Association*, 2000; 284: 2489–2494 (PMID 11074779).

16. Travis SS, Bernard M, Dixon S, McAuley WJ, Loving G, McClanahan L. Obstacles to palliation and end-of-life care in a long-term care facility. *Gerontologist* 2002; 42: 342–349 (PMID 12040136).

17. Hoffman DE, Tarzian AJ. Dying in America—an examination of policies that deter adequate end-of-life care in nursing homes. *Journal of Law, Medicine and Ethics* 2005; 33, no. 2 (abstract). Available at ssrn.com/abstract=733625 (accessed June 17, 2007).

18. Kayser-Jones J, Schell E, Lyons W, Kris AE, Chan J, Beard RL. Factors that influence end-of-life care in nursing homes: the physical environment, inadequate staffing and lack of supervision. *Gerontologist* 2003; 43, Spec No. 2:76–84 (PMID 12711727).

19. Cassarett D, Karlawish J, Morales K, Crowley R, Mirsch T, Asch DA. Improving the use of hospice services in nursing homes: a randomized controlled trial. *Journal of the American Medical Association* 2005; 294: 211–217 (PMID 16014595).

20. Hoffmann DE, Tarzian DJ. Dying in America: An examination of policies that deter adequate end-of-life care in nursing homes. *Journal of Law, Medicine and Ethics* 2005:33 (No. 2) available at http://ssrn.com/abstract=73365 (accessed June 17, 2007).

21. Holahan J, Weil A. Toward real Medicaid reform. *Health Affairs* 2007; 26: w254–w270 (PMID 17322276).

Chapter 7

1. Gillick MR. Rethinking the central dogma of palliative care. *Journal of Palliative Medicine* 2005; 8: 909–913 (PMID 16238502).

2. Grief is a journey too. Perspective section, *Chicago Tribune*, section 2, p. 3, November 26, 2006.

3. Super. Ct. Civ. Action No. 92-4820, Suffolk Co., Mass. verdict, 21 April 1995. See also Capron AM. *AT law: abandoning a waning life. Hastings Center Report* 1995; 25: 24–26, p. 26 (PMID 7591722).

4. See www.ampainsoc.org/advocacy/treatment.htm (accessed March 2, 2007).

5. Gordon DB, Dahl JL, Miaskowski C, McCarberg B, et al. American Pain Society recommendations for improving the quality of acute and cancer pain management: American Pain Society quality of care task force. *Archives of Internal Medicine* 2005; 165: 1574–1580 (PMID 16043674).

6. See www.crha-health.ab.ca/clin/cme/cpg/palliativesedation1999.pdf (accessed March 7, 2007).

7. Burt RA. The Supreme Court speaks—not assisted suicide but a constitutional right to palliative care. *New England Journal of Medicine* 1997; 337: 1234–1236 (PMID 9337388).

8. See en.wikipedia.org/wiki/Elisabeth_K%C3%Bcbler-Ross.

9. Hoffmann RL. The evolution of hospice in America: nursing's role in the movement. *Journal of Gerontological Nursing* 2005; 31: 26–34 (PMID 16047957).

10. Campbell DE, Lynn J, Louis TA, Shugarman LR. Medicare program expenditures associated with hospice use. *Annals of Internal Medicine* 2004; 140: 269–277 (PMID 14970150).

11. Lubitz JD, Riley GF. Trends in Medicare payments in the last year of life. *New England Journal of Medicine* 1993; 328: 1092–1096 (PMID 8455667).

12. Hoover DR, Crystal S, Kumar R, Sambamoorthi U, Cantor JC. Medical expenditures during the last year of life: findings from the 1992–1996 Medicare beneficiary survey. *Health Services Research* 2002; 37: 1625–1642 (PMID 12546289).

13. Weiss SC Editor's note. Economics, ethics, and end-of-life care. *Journal of the American Medical Association* 1999; 282: 2076 (PMID 10591392).

14. Brody H, Campbell ML, Faber-Langendoen K, Ogle KS. Sounding board: Withdrawing intensive life-sustaining treatment—recommendations for compassionate clinical management. *New England Journal of Medicine* 1997; 336: 652–657 (PMID 9032053).

15. Fox E, Landrum-McNiff K, Zhoug Z, Dawson NV, Wu AW, Lynn J. Evaluation of prognostic criteria for determining hospice eligibility in patients with advanced lung, heart or liver disease. Support Investigators. Study to understand prognoses and preferences for outcomes and risks of treatments. *Journal of the American Medical Association* 1999; 282: 1638–1645 (PMID 10553790).

Chapter 10

1. Ginsburg PB, Berenson RA. Revising Medicare's physician fee schedule—much activity, little change. *New England Journal of Medicine* 2007; 356: 1201–1203 (PMID 17377156).

2. See www.elderweb.com/home/taxonomy/term/6370.

3. See www.ahca.org/brief/seidmanstudy0606.pdf.

4. Popp RL, Lorell BH, Stone GW, et al. An outline for public registration of clinical trials evaluating medical devices. *Journal of the American College of Cardiology* 2006; 47: 1518–1521 (PMID 16630985).

5. Mitka M. Cardiologists get wake-up call on stents. *Journal of the American Medical Association* 2007; 297: 1967–1968 (PMID 17488954).

6. See healthsignals.typepad.com/newyork/2005/06/the argument ag.html (accessed April 5, 2007).

7. *Long-term care: aging baby boom generation will increase demand and burden on federal and state budgets.* Statement of David M. Walker, Comptroller General of the United States, before the Special Committee on Aging, U.S. Senate. U.S. General Accounting Office Report, March 21, 2002.

8. Mechanic D. *The truth about health care: why reform is not working in America.* New Brunswick, N.J.: Rutgers University Press, 2006.

9. What is behind HRSA's projected supply, demand, and shortage of registered Nurses? Health Resources and Services Administration (HRSA). September 2004, pp. 10–12.

10. See en.eikipedia.org/wiki/pharmaceutical (accessed April 4, 2007).

11. Donohue JM, Cevasco M, Rosenthal MB. A decade of direct-to-consumer advertising of prescription drugs. *New England Journal of Medicine* 2007; 357: 673–681. (PMID 17699817).

12. http://familiesusa.org/404/html. Prescription drugs, drug industry, the choice: Healthcare for people or drug industry profits, key findings.

13. See http://www.aflcio.org/about aflcio/magazine/0503_bigfix.cfm (accessed December 26, 2007).

14. http://www.nybooks.com/articles/17244.

15. Baim DS, Donovan A, Smith J, Briefs N, Geoffrion R, Feigal D, Kaplan AV. Medical device development: managing conflicts of interest encountered by physicians. *Catheterization and Cardiovascular Interventions* 2007; 69: 655–664 (PMID 17390305).

16. Popp RL, Covell BH, Stone GW, et al. An outline for public registration of clinical trials evaluating medical devices. *Journal of the American College of Cardiology* 2006; 47: 1518–1521 (PMID 16630985).

17. Boden WE, O'Rourke, Koon KK, Hartigan PM, et al. Optimal medical therapy with or without PCI for stable coronary disease. *New England Journal of Medicine* 2007; 356: 1503–1516 (PMID 17387127). See also Hochman JS, Steg PG. Does preventive PCI work? Editorial. *New England Journal of Medicine* 2007; 356:1572–1574 (PMID 17387128).

18. Coyne DW. Use of epoetin in chronic renal failure. *Journal of the American Medical Association* 2007; 297: 1713–1716 (PMID 17440149).

Glossary

Acute care facility. A facility, generally a hospital, that provides curative care for illness or injury.

Acute illness. A recent illness with rapid onset and usually a short course, such as an earache or the flu.

ADA. A 1990 federal law that forbids discrimination against persons who are disabled.

Advance directive. Generally a written decision with instructions and preferences for medical treatment. There may also be a designation of a person to make decisions should the patient be unable to do so.

Alzheimer's disease. a progressive form of dementia. The first symptoms are impaired memory, which is followed by impaired thought and speech, and finally complete helplessness and lack of awareness or recognition of surroundings.

Americans with Disabilities Act (ADA). A 1990 federal law that forbids discrimination against persons who are disabled.

Angiogram. An X-ray of blood vessels in which the vessels are outlined by a dye injected before the procedure.

Atherosclerosis. Clogging, narrowing, and hardening of the body's large arteries and medium-sized blood vessels. It can lead to stroke, heart attack, eye problems, and kidney problems.

Arteriosclerosis. A normal consequence of aging where the arterial walls gradually thicken, arterial fibers decline, and the arteries become stiff.

Baby boomers. Those born between 1946 and 1964.

Blood flow scan. Measures blood flow to a particular part of the body, especially the brain.

Brain death. The total and permanent loss of all brain function (both cerebral cortex and brainstem stem) that is one of the medical and legal determinations of death.

Brainstem stem. The brainstem stem, at the base of the brain, carries out "primitive functions," such as breathing, swallowing, and blood pressure. Is needed along with the cerebral cortex for wakefulness.

Cancer. A malignant growth or tumor caused by abnormal and uncontrolled cell division that may spread to other parts of the body through the lymphatic system or the blood stream.

Cardiologist. A physician who is a heart specialist.

Cardiopulmonary resuscitation (CPR). A method of artificial breathing and circulation, usually administered by a CPR-certified responder when the natural heart action and breathing have stopped. Artificial rescue breaths and chest compressions are used. In some cases (full code status), a defibrillator may be used to electrically shock the heart back into action.

Cardioversion. Applying electrical shock to the chest to change an abnormal heartbeat into a normal one.

Cardioverter defibrillator. Electronic devices implanted in the patient's chest that automatically cardiovert or defibrillate (deliver a shock to the patient's heart) when triggered by abnormal heart rate or patterns.

Cellulitis. A spreading bacterial infection just below the skin surface most commonly caused by *Streptococcus pyogenes* that creates acute inflammation.

Cerebral cortex. The part of the brain capable of thinking, planning, communication, memory, and problem solving. It is the picture that comes to mind when we think of the "brain," and is the place where our alertness and humanness reside.

Cerebral palsy. A general term for a group of permanent brain injuries that affect an infant in the womb, during birth, or in the months following birth. Cerebral palsy patients may have limited motor skills, speech difficulties, learning disabilities, or other problems.

Chronic illness. Diseases of slow progression and long duration such as arthritis, cardiac disorders, emphysema, etc.

Chronic obstructive pulmonary disease (COPD). A progressive lung disease process characterized by difficulty breathing, wheezing, and a chronic cough. Complications include bronchitis, pneumonia, and lung cancer.

Cirrhosis. A condition in which the liver becomes scarred and fibrous (scar cells replace liver cells), thus reducing its ability to function.

Coma. A coma is a profound or deep state of unconsciousness. An individual in a state of coma is alive but unable to move or respond to his or her environment. Coma may occur as a complication of an underlying illness, or as a result of injuries, such as head trauma.

Comorbidity. The presence of coexisting or additional conditions or diseases besides the initial diagnosis that may effect treatment outcome or patient survival.

Congestive heart failure. Heart failure caused by loss of pumping power by the heart, resulting in fluids collecting in the body. It can be treated by drugs and in some cases, by surgery.

Contagious disease. A disease that is easily passed from one person to another.

COPD – Chronic obstructive pulmonary disease. A progressive lung disease process characterized by difficulty breathing, wheezing, and a chronic cough. Complications include bronchitis, pneumonia, and lung cancer.

Critical care unit. A section of a hospital providing greater than ordinary medical care and observation to people in a critical or unstable condition.

Decubitii. Severe skin breakdown, such as bedsores. Decubitii are common in bed-ridden patients, and are difficult to resolve or to control the spread.

Defibrillator. A device used to correct a dangerously abnormal heart rhythm, usually ventricular fibrillation, or to restart a heart that has stopped beating.

Dementia. The loss of intellectual functions (such as thinking, remembering, and reasoning) of sufficient severity to interfere with a person's daily functioning. Dementia is irreversible when caused by disease or injury but may be reversible when caused by drugs, alcohol, hormone or vitamin imbalances, or depression.

Diabetes. A chronic health condition associated with higher than normal levels of sugar in the blood. In type 1 (insulin-dependent) diabetes, there is no insulin or not enough of it. In type 2 diabetes, there is generally enough insulin, but the cells are not normally sensitive to its action.

Diagnostic-related groups (DRGs). DRGs are patient classification systems that group patients according to diagnosis and treatment for the purpose of setting uniform payment rates for hospital care. The goal is more cost-effective care.

Dialysis. The process of cleaning wastes from the blood artificially with special equipment when the kidneys are unable to do so.

Disability. A physical or mental condition which inhibits or prevents normal daily function.

Do not resuscitate order (DNR). An order dictating that an individual does not desire resuscitative measures in the case of failed breathing or cardiac arrest.

Electroencephalogram (EEG). A test that measures brain waves.

Emphysema. A chronic, irreversible disease of the lungs.

Epilepsy. A disorder of the brain that results in recurrent, unprovoked seizures.

Full code status. A directive that all measures of resuscitation be undertaken if a patient suffers respiratory or cardiac arrest.

Gastrostomy tube. A tube inserted into the body of a patient who cannot take nutrition and fluids orally.

Gross domestic product (GDP). The total value of goods and services produced by a nation.

Hospice. Healthcare services providing medical care and support services such as counseling to terminally ill people and their families.

Hospitalist. A physician who practices general internal medicine and practices only in hospitals, taking care of other physicians' patients.

Intensive Care Unit (ICU). A section of a hospital providing greater than ordinary medical care and observation to people in a critical or unstable condition.

Intubation. The procedure of inserting a tube into the trachea of a patient who is not breathing.

Kidney failure. A condition in which the kidneys fail to function properly or cease functioning altogether.

Life support. Procedures designed to keep a patient alive when certain bodily functions are impaired, such as placing a patient on a ventilator when they cannot breathe on their own.

Medicaid. Federally funded health insurance for the poor and disabled regardless of their age.

Medicare. Federally funded health insurance program for people sixty-five years or older.

Morbidity. An undesired condition or outcome. In medical terms, a disease or abnormal physical condition that compromises health.

Multiple infarct dementia. dementia caused by a series of small strokes.

Myocardial infarction. Heart attack.

Nephrologist. A physician specializing in kidney function and disorders.

Nursing home. A healthcare facility, generally separate from a hospital that provides various types of care depending on need. They may provide short- or long-term care, physical therapy, skilled nursing care for specific patient populations such as those with severe mental conditions, and intermediate care such as the transition from an acute care hospital to assisted living or home care. There are also custodial care facilities that provide services to the elderly that enable them to remain at home.

Palliative care. Care that provides relief from symptoms and pain, but has no curative action.

Palliative education assessment tool for medical education (PEAT). A curriculum developed to teach palliative care techniques in medical schools.

Palliative surgery. Surgery that provides relief from symptoms, but does not necessarily have a curative effect.

Patient autonomy. The right of patients to make decisions regarding their healthcare, particularly the right to refuse treatment, and to create advance directives regarding their care at the end of life.

Patient Self-Determination Act (PSDA). A law passed by Congress in 1990 that stated that patients have the right under state law to create advance directives stipulating what they wish done in an end-of-life situation.

Persistent vegetative state. Individuals in such a state have lost their thinking abilities and awareness of their surroundings usually after loss of oxygen to the brain through injury or some other physical event. They retain noncognitive function and normal sleep patterns. Even though those in a persistent vegetative state lose their higher brain functions, other key functions such as breathing and circulation remain relatively intact. Spontaneous movements may occur, and the eyes may open in response to external stimuli. They may even occasionally grimace, cry, or laugh. Although individuals in a persistent vegetative state may appear somewhat physically normal, they do not have consciousness thus cannot think, are unaware of their surroundings, and cannot communicate. Before the advent of artificial nutrition and other supportive measures, they did not survive.

Primary care. Basic or general healthcare focused on the point at which a patient ideally first seeks assistance from the medical care system. Primary care physicians were once referred to as "the family doctor."

Renal failure. A condition in which the kidneys fail to function properly, or cease functioning altogether.

Sepsis. Bacteria in the blood causing systemic infection.

Specialty hospitals. Private hospitals, often physician-owned, that specialize in a single area of medicine, such as ventilators, cardiac procedures, orthopedic procedures, and ophthalmology procedures such as cataract surgeries.

Stent. A device placed in a body structure (such as a blood vessel or the gastrointestinal tract) to provide support and keep the structure open.

Stroke. The sudden death of some brain cells due to a lack of oxygen when the blood flow to the brain is impaired by blockage or rupture of an artery to the brain.

Teaching hospital. A hospital affiliated with or part of a medical school where students can gain firsthand experience in a hospital.

Terminal illness. A condition that is incurable and irreversible where the only outcome is death.

Terminal sedation. Administration of sedating and pain-relieving drugs at the end of a patient's life to control extreme suffering.

Vasculitis. Inflamed blood vessels.

Ventilator. A mechanical device to facilitate breathing in persons with impaired lung or diaphragm function, or patients who cannot breathe on their own.

Index

About the Authors

BENJAMIN BROWN, M.D. is a family doctor in a community-based primary care center in rural Central Virginia. He includes his long-term interest in acupuncture in his practice. During off hours, he enjoys his family while walking in the mountains, canoeing the rivers, and landscaping their home.

KENNETH A. FISHER, M.D. is a nephrology consultant for the Borgess and Bronson Hospitals in Kalamazoo, Michigan. For over forty years, he has served in a variety of clinical, teaching, and research positions. He has written dozens of scientific and policy articles in such publications as *Clinical Nephrology*, *American Journal of Physiology*, *American Journal of Medicine*, and *American Journal of Obstetrics and Gynecology*.

LINDSAY E. ROCKWELL, D.O. is a hematologist and oncologist in private practice in Northampton, Massachusetts. She is the Director of Integrative Oncology at Cooley-Dickinson Hospital and is involved in numerous research endeavors examining the role of complementary medicine for the oncology patient. She has been published in the *Journal of Clinical Oncology*, presents at oncology conferences, and has a special interest in palliative care as well as women's issues in the context of cancer care.

MISSY SCOTT, a former broadcast journalist, is a freelance writer and instructional designer. She writes courseware and supporting materials for teachers in colleges, universities, and healthcare training schools.